THE ABA PROGRAM COMPANION

Organizing Quality Programs for Children with Autism and PDD

J. Tyler Fovel, M.A.,
Board Certified Behavior Analyst™

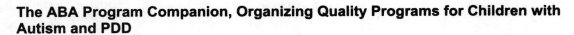

The ABA Program Companion, Organizing Quality Programs for Children with Autism and PDD

The Consultant's Companion Curriculum Development Software

Published by: DRL Books, Inc.
12 West 18th Street, Suite 3E
New York, New York 10011
Phone: (800) 853-1057
Fax: (212) 206-9329
www.drlbooks.com

Permission is gratefully acknowledged to use material from the curriculum contained in *A Work in Progress,* copyright © 1999, Autism Partnership. All rights reserved.

Library of Congress Control Number: 2002108149
ISBN Number: 978-0966-5266-7-7

Printed in the United States of America

To Jan, who loves children and teaching—in that order.

TABLE OF CONTENTS

Chapter 1

Chapter 2

Chapter 3

Chapter 4

Chapter 5

INCIDENTAL TEACHING 73

Chapter 6

SOCIAL INTERACTION AND INTEGRATION................................. 82

Chapter 7

Chapter 8

Chapter 9

Chapter 10

Appendix

Teaching Evaluation Checklist
Typical Instructions for Preschoolers and Kindergarteners
Discrete trials data sheet
Stimulus list
Mand list
Potential reinforcer list
Student schedule form
Incidental language data sheet
Incidental teaching form
Probe data sheet
Curriculum form
Mastered list form

Preface

Brad is Beginning an ABA Program

Brad is approaching his third birthday and his parents are trying to get him started in an ABA program. They have agreed with their local school district that an ABA program would best serve Brad's needs and that Brad will receive a 30 hour per week program in the local school with an individual paraprofessional implementing the program under the supervision of a special education teacher. The school district has contracted with a regional center-based ABA program to provide ongoing training and consultation. School district administrators are anxious to provide an appropriate program for Brad but they are inexperienced in ABA and are looking to the consultants to develop a systematic strategy that addresses assessment, training, program development, and evaluation. Everyone involved understands that a great deal of effort and resources will be required over a sustained period of time but their main concern is to provide a successful, high-quality program. The effort will be made by a number of personnel—teachers, paraprofessional, parents, consultants, related-service providers, and administrators—and it will take time. However, the educational team is committed to making the program work and is looking forward to the challenge.

What This Manual is—

This manual is specifically designed to be used as a resource by educational teams like Brad's, especially special educators and program coordinators, working to help organize and implement ABA programs. Read this manual if you are setting up an ABA program, want to improve your knowledge of ABA, or just want some ideas to improve an existing ABA program. Despite all that has been written in the field of autism, there is still a pressing need to provide teams with practical guidance on establishing programs with a consistent system of development, implementation, and review. That is the present focus. Obviously, as the field has become more widely known and popular, parents and educators are increasingly interested in setting up new programs. Consequently, the need for a straightforward, comprehensive, and organized approach is more important than ever.

What This Manual is not—

This manual does not contain a curriculum. Nor is there information on the nature and diagnosis of autism, the efficacy of ABA, or discussion of every important topic relating to treatment. Other sources will be necessary to provide information on topics not covered or where additional detail may be desired. Some of these sources are provided at the end of each chapter.

This manual is not at all sufficient as a replacement for a qualified consultant or program coordinator. The Association for Behavior Analysis has established requirements for education, experience, and certification of *Board Certified Behavior Analysts™*. In addition, a subgroup of the ABA, the Special Interest Group (SIG) for autism has published specifications for those wishing to be considered qualified ABA consultants. All educational teams should become aware of these two sets of skills necessary for persons claiming to be ABA consultants. On the Internet, see:

http://www.wmich.edu/aba.

Forms, Reports and Software

The organizational methodology contained in this manual including forms, evaluations, checklists, etc. is based on practical experience and represents *one way* to organize programs. While the methods presented have proven consistent and useful in the author's experience with a number of educational teams, it should be recognized that alternative systems or ideas could also be productive. In order to produce the curriculum reports shown in the illustrations and organize the process of curriculum goal development, a free software program is included on the CD-ROM that accompanies this manual. This is a time-saving way of organizing and documenting a student's curriculum for Windows™ based computers. Instructions on installing and using the software are included in Chapter 10 and on the CD. However, there is no reason why these reports could not be made using other databases or a word processor.

Use of Materials

Since the purpose of this manual is to provide teams with tools to help organize educational programs, permission is granted to photocopy and modify the forms presented. In addition, the various chapters and materials may be photocopied for clinical, non-commercial use as long as the copyright notice is not removed. The reproduction of the manual as a whole or the reproduction of any portion of this manual for resale is not permitted.

How to Use This Manual

Here are some hints for getting the most out of this manual:

The materials included can be used with or adapted for school, center, or home-based programs. The sections on program development and organization, and the associated forms, when paired with a good curriculum, are usually sufficient to create a well-structured, comprehensive and individualized plan. The chapters on basic behavior analysis can be presented to new teaching personnel as introductions to the field and as a foundation for the more specific sections on discrete trial teaching, teaching in other formats, inclusion, etc. Note that there are focus questions at the end of each chapter that can help identify important concepts.

Some readers will be familiar with many of the clinical concepts presented. Others will be encountering them for the first time. Browsing through the manual once all the way through will help you to become familiar with the scope and presentation style of the material so that you can decide how best it will be of use to you (i.e., what forms you will use, what procedures you will follow, what trainings you will conduct, etc.). After reading a chapter, if you still have questions, you may want to do some further reading to become comfortable with an area before proceeding. Remember, however, that some topics are further developed in succeeding chapters and a careful reading of the book all the way through from the beginning will yield the maximum benefit.

Carefully go over the required basic competencies for paraprofessionals and the Program Audit (Part IV) *before* you start your program or, at least, as soon as possible. This will help you to become oriented towards the *product* of your efforts—setting up a quality program.

What's on the CD?

The accompanying CD-ROM contains more material designed to help you set up your program. There are:

- electronic versions of forms
- a beta-version of *The Consultant's Companion* software program for Windows™

Feel free to contribute comments and suggestions and help make the manual better:

E-Mail: tfovel@strategic-alternatives.com
U.S. Mail to: Tyler Fovel, Strategic Alternatives, 15 Deerfield Road, Medway, Massachusetts, 02053
Web: http://strategic-alternatives.com

Acknowledgements

This manual is dedicated to the parents of children with autism and PDD for whom I have worked. Through their love, determination, and dedication to their children they have inspired me both professionally and personally to strive for greater excellence. Respect for their privacy prevents me from mentioning their names but I cannot begin to articulate the lessons I have learned in daily contact with them and I hope I can give back even a fraction of what I have gained. I would also like to thank the many people who have contributed directly to this project. Encouragement from Karen Gould and Julie Azuma helped launch a serious rewrite of the first draft. Myrna Libby, Shelagh Conway, Katie Vincenzo, Bridgett Zawoy, Heather Baker, Maryanne Harmuth, and Melissa Tott read drafts and gave me valuable feedback. Lisa Selznick read the manuscript twice and gave wonderfully detailed and helpful editorial advice. Meghan Fovel meticulously proofed the final copy. Thanks are also due to the staff at LEARN ABA in East Lyme, Connecticut for their enthusiasm and support including Jody Lefkowitz, Abby Dolliver, Vicki Wolfe, Erica Andresen, and Heather Baker. Finally, I would like to thank my wife Jan for always having just the right insight or comment when needed. Living with a master teacher has its benefits. Her wisdom, sensitivity, and encouragement helped me more than she realizes but most of all she shared with me the secrets of the world of children and teachers.

Introduction

THE ANATOMY OF AN ABA PROGRAM

ABA programs vary considerably but, like good educational programs in general, they have certain characteristics that form the core of everything else that they do. These core characteristics are listed below. Good ABA programs implement these characteristics explicitly and systematically, often far more than other program models, with a firm commitment to objective, data-driven analysis of behavior and teaching strategies.

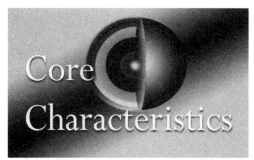

Establish a Baseline of Skills

Observation and repeated measurement of the student's baseline level of skills is accomplished early in the intake process using objective methods. The student's repertoire is compared skill by skill to the program's developmental curriculum, noting mastered skills, those partially mastered, and those that are not yet appropriate. Student preferences and behavior issues are also evaluated.

Specify an Appropriate Curriculum

Curriculum is specified in multiple areas relevant to the student's age, strengths and needs. Early curriculum usually includes an emphasis on language, social skills, play, and "learning-to-learn" skills. Early skill development provides the prerequisites for later acquisition of more complex skills and careful attention is paid to proper sequencing of programs. The curriculum is implemented in various settings appropriate to the student's developmental needs and abilities with strong emphasis on generalization of skills to the natural environment.

Give Frequent Learning Opportunities

Every minute of the student's day counts. Learning activities are structured to maximize the opportunity of the student to engage in new behavior that will be reinforced in multiple settings throughout the day. A paraprofessional is usually assigned to the student, giving the educational team important additional resources. The paraprofessional implements the student's schedule and curriculum as designed by the

ABA consultant and educational team. Skills are broken down into simple parts and students are presented with multiple opportunities to practice the skills, followed by meaningful and motivating rewards for good work.

Continuously Evaluate Progress

One hallmark of an ABA program is to continuously evaluate the performance and progress of the student through data collection and graphing. Daily data is collected on the student's performance in all areas and compared to established criteria for advancement. Under supervision, the paraprofessional moves the student forward as soon as the criteria is reached, minimizing delay and boredom. Lack of progress is easily identified in the data, which propels early revision of unproductive methodology.

Part 1: Basic Training

UNDERSTANDING BEHAVIOR - Fundamental Aspects of Teaching

It is important that teachers, paraprofessionals, and parents carrying out programs understand *how* to teach in addition to *what* should be taught; developing a keen understanding of behavior and its causes is vital in establishing this awareness. Two central topics in applied behavior analysis will be introduced first that will set the scene for more specific training later.

1. Changing behavior through consequences
2. Changing behavior by arranging antecedent conditions

Chapter 1

USING CONSEQUENCES TO CHANGE BEHAVIOR

Introduction: Observing and Describing Behavior

Some readers may wonder what is meant by the word *behavior*. According to a prominent textbook on behavior analysis, a behavior is:

> "…an organism's interaction with its environment that is characterized by detectable [movement] in space through time of some part of the organism …that results in a measurable change in the environment."

> (Johnston & Pennypacker, 1993, P. 23.)

A key thought in this definition is that behavior is an *observable movement* by the organism. Descriptions of behavior that contain the most useful information, from the standpoint of behavior analysis and teaching, use descriptions that are observable and measurable. Everyday language is filled with imprecise speech that often leads to incorrect interpretations and confusion about behavior. We might say that a person was "unhappy" earlier in the day even though all that was observed was an intense look on the person's face during a study time. A child who has tantrums might be described as "angry" at his teachers or "rebellious." When motives or internal emotional states are assigned to behavior a biased interpretation of the situation is imposed on those exposed only to an interpretation, not the raw facts. Furthermore, such descriptions are difficult to talk about consistently. How often is the student "unhappy?" Even a close observer may not consistently identify behavior that is described so imprecisely.

Consider the following items from our fictitious newspaper *The Non-Behavioral Daily Times*. On page 1 of the City & Region section, under Lost & Found, an article advertising for the return of a lost cat is placed: "*Please look out for Buffy, our family cat*. She was lost yesterday. She is loving, playful, curious, and a real rascal. If found, please call 456-8934." Do you think the family will see that cat again?

On the same page this news item is found: "The State Bank was robbed yesterday by five men who got away with $50,000. Witnesses described the men as suspicious-acting, fearful, aggressive, hostile, cruel, and unintelligent. Police are investigating." Further down on the page in a related article: "Following witness descriptions, police brought in 316 men for questioning in connection with the robbery of the State Bank..." Let's hope that someone confesses! Objective and observable descriptions are more reliable. Using words that describe the actions or form of the behavior and avoiding interpretations or *inferred mental states* leads to more productive discussions and a clearer understanding of what is going on.

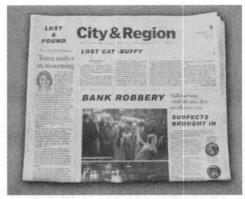

Attributes of Behavior

Using words that describe observable actions rather than inferred mental states or interpretations is the first big step towards the scientific study of behavior. If the behavior is objectively described its occurrence can be studied and important information learned. Four aspects of the occurrence of behavior can be especially useful: *frequency, duration, latency, and intensity.*

- *Frequency* refers to the number of times a behavior occurs during a particular time period.
- *Duration* refers to how long a particular behavior lasts.
- *Latency* refers to how much time passes between a prompt or initial event of some kind and the occurrence of the behavior.
- *Intensity* refers to the force with which a behavior occurs.

Let's look at an example at the baseball park. Baseball (and other sports) fans seem to be obsessed with measuring behavior of all types. They measure the *frequency* of many things including the number of pitches thrown, number of strikes, balls, singles, doubles, home runs, wins, and losses. Sports fans also measure the *duration* of the game or even the duration of the "hang time" of a jumper in basketball (length of time in the air). *Latency* is measured when we measure how much time elapses between gaining possession of the ball and scoring (football). *Intensity* could be measured in the force of a punch (boxing). Sometimes intensity is estimated or inferred from the results of the behavior like measuring the distance of travel of the baseball off the bat or the speed of the baseball thrown.

Graphs

Collecting objective information on behavior like frequency, duration, latency, or intensity gives us an excellent basis for making decisions about the nature and causes of behavior. The numbers by themselves are helpful but there are ways to translate raw numbers into a display that helps viewers to judge what is happening to the behavior over time. Data that has been collected over several days is presented in a table below. Try and judge what is happening to the values over the course of days. What is the approximate middle value? How variable is the data from day to day? Answers to these questions are not immediately obvious from looking at the table.

Data Table										
Date:	3/1/02	3/2/02	3/3/02	3/4/02	3/5/02	3/6/02	3/7/02	3/8/02	3/9/02	3/10/02
Value:	10	20	15	30	20	30	26	30	38	31

Graphs play an important role in behavior analysis. Measurements of a behavior at any point in time capture only a snapshot of the behavior but not how that behavior is changing over time. If we make multiple measurements at regular time intervals we can display each of these measurements as a point on a graph.

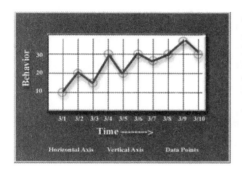

Time is usually displayed on the *horizontal axis*, increasing from left to right. The measure of the behavior (frequency, duration, etc.) is then displayed on the *vertical axis*. Each measurement is plotted on the graph as a *data point*, at the intersection of the time value and the behavior value.

Graphs are particularly useful for a number of things including:

- helping to detect trends in the data
- visualizing the values of a large amount of data at one time
- comparing one group of data points with another

The Timeline of Behavior

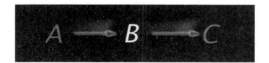

The graphic above, called here a *Timeline of Behavior*, diagrams the basic events involved in behavior change. As indicated by the arrows, time moves from left to right. Whenever we look at teaching or behavior change in general it's helpful to remember this diagram. *Antecedents* precede *Behavior* followed by *Consequences;* the history of relationships between these three events determines when a specific behavior occurs and how often. *History* means the times in the past where a particular behavior occurred in the presence of certain people, things, or places (antecedents) and when the behavior was followed by other events (consequences). It is these events in time that form the history of a particular behavior with the conditions under which it comes to occur.

Examples of Consequences

- Ice cream is a treat that some children hope for. If it reliably follows a particular behavior (consequence), we might expect more of the behavior in the future.
- A mom's scolding reaction (consequence) to her son's premature taste of cake before dinner is designed to decrease the probability that it will happen in the future.
- Compliments and praise (consequences) following appropriate behavior often go a long way towards ensuring that the behavior occurs again.

In these examples an occurrence of behavior is followed by a particular consequence, affecting the future probability of occurrence of the behavior. This is what is meant by the terms *history of reinforcement* or *history of punishment*. Consistently providing certain types of consequences to specific behaviors will strengthen or weaken the probability of occurrence of a behavior over time.

Examples of consequences designed to increase behavior in a classroom might include:

- Complimenting a child when he uses a creative word
- Awarding a star or points for children who are helpful or kind to each other in class
- Awarding prizes for creative science projects

Examples of attempting to *decrease* behavior with consequences might include:

- Taking away five minutes of recess because the class was disruptive
- Prompting a child to sit in the time out chair for 2 minutes after she ran in class during free play
- Reprimanding a student for not completing his homework

Contingencies

The procedures of using consequences and their effects on behavior can be diagrammed. In the table below a *stimulus* is defined as some event or object in a person's environment. The stimulus is delivered immediately after the occurrence of a particular behavior. This is called a *contingency*. A contingency is a rule: "If you do behavior X, consequence Y will occur. Generally speaking, there are four possible ways (contingencies) of using consequences that result in changes in behavior. These procedures are named.

1. When you *add* a stimulus after a behavior and the frequency of the behavior tends to *increase,* the procedure is called *positive reinforcement*.

2. When you *take away* a stimulus after a behavior and the frequency of the behavior tends to *increase,* the procedure is called *negative reinforcement.*

3. When you *add* a stimulus after a behavior and the frequency of the behavior tends to *decrease*, the procedure is called *punishment* (or *type 1 punishment*).

4. When you *take away* a stimulus after a behavior and the frequency of the behavior tends to *decrease,* the procedure is called *time out* (or *type II punishment*).

You may have noticed that the procedure is only named *after* the change in behavior is observed. For example, adding a stimulus after a behavior is called positive reinforcement only if the behavior tends to increase in the future. In the same way, delivering candy for correct answers is called positive reinforcement if the correct answers tend to increase. Behavior analysts refer to the procedures as being defined by *operation* and *function*. Operation refers to the addition or withdrawal of a stimulus while function refers to the effect of the operation on the future probability of occurrence of the behavior.

Table of Consequence-Based Procedures (Contingencies)

Operation	Function	
(1) When you...	**(2)...and the behavior**	
	Increases (+)	Decreases (-)
	THE PROCEDURE IS CALLED:	
Add a stimulus (+)	Positive Reinforcement	Type I Punishment
Take away a stimulus (-)	Negative Reinforcement	Time Out or Type II Punishment

Examples of positive reinforcement are usually easy to understand. Negative reinforcement, however, is often misunderstood and further explanation may be helpful. According to definition, negative reinforcement occurs when a stimulus is *withdrawn* following a behavior and the behavior tends to *increase*. This phenomenon is also called *escape*. Imagine an unpleasantly loud noise that constantly sounds in a room. If we can simply move to a panel of switches (like an alarm panel) and flip a switch to turn the sound off, negative reinforcement (or escape) has probably occurred. The behavior of flipping the switch is most likely strengthened each time the noise sounds because it results in turning off the unpleasant noise. Often the stimuli that are taken away in negative reinforcement are unpleasant or *aversive stimuli*. When a stimulus consistently follows behavior and the behavior decreases the definition of *punishment* (type I) is met. Some aversive stimuli are obvious (e.g., reprimands or painful physical stimuli) but sometimes more subtle events like "constructive feedback" or critical looks can punish and decrease behavior.

Time out (also called *Type II punishment*) uses a different method to decrease behavior. In this procedure a stimulus is *taken away* resulting in a decrease in the future probability of occurrence of the behavior. Penalties fall into this category. If we take away money or privileges based on the occurrence of a behavior and the behavior decreases, time out has occurred. Possibly another scenario is a more familiar representation of the concept. If a child is playing and slaps another child, the caregiver may have the child sit down for a period of time before resuming play. If the behavior of slapping decreases in the future, this would also be called time out because the opportunity to play is taken away contingent on the behavior.

Using Positive Reinforcement

Contingencies are powerful techniques for changing behavior, especially using positive reinforcement. *"Catch the child being good!"* is old and appropriate advice to teachers. Throughout the child's day, in every setting, appropriate behavior can be increased by reinforcing it meaningfully. Of course, this means becoming alert to the child's good behavior when, so often, we are attuned to the bad. Nevertheless, it is well worth the effort and creates a positive atmosphere.

We need not wait for perfect behavior in order to reinforce a child. We may develop a plan of reinforcing *successive approximations* to the ultimate target behavior. Given a child who is constantly fidgeting we may not want to wait for a five full minutes of quiet behavior to reinforce but require only 15 seconds at first. As the occasions of sitting quietly for 15 seconds increase we may revise our requirement to 30 seconds followed by 45 seconds, etc. In this way we gradually *shape* the behavior into what we want to see.

Discovering Effective Reinforcers

Merely following target behaviors with events that we *presume* to be reinforcing is not the best way to ensure an increase in the behaviors. The person's unique desires, needs, and history determine the effectiveness of stimuli as reinforcers. Reinforcers can only be discovered through observation and experimentation. Moreover, what is reinforcing at one moment may not be reinforcing at another. Therefore, a large list of effective stimuli that can, potentially, serve as reinforcers is crucial to the development of a good educational program.

Reinforcing stimuli are not limited to praise and candy. The particular quality or reinforcing dimension of a stimulus can appeal to any sense as seen in the table below.

Reinforcing Dimension of Stimulus	Examples
Social	Being with a person, eye-contact, smiles, interactive games, talking to a person, parties, winning
Gustatory	(Taste or consumption-related) pizza, Burger King, candy, soda, salty, swallowing, chewing
Auditory	Music, singing, novel sounds
Visual	Colors, bright lights, motion pictures, art, attractive people
Tactile	Hugs, roughhousing, tickling, massage, cool breeze on a hot day, vibration, warm blanket
Proprioceptive	Exercising, throwing a ball, stretching, bowling
Olfactory	Perfume, flowers, food aromas
Vestibular	Rocking, amusement park rides, swings, rides in vehicles, bicycle riding, running, trampolines

Limitations of Sole Use of Consequences

As part of our arsenal of behavior change techniques, consequences can be quite effective. However, in order for reinforcers to be delivered properly, a suitable behavior must occur. This may be difficult when those delivering reinforcers are not present constantly to see the behavior when it does occur. If target behaviors for increase occur rarely, it may be nearly impossible to reliably provide reinforcing consequences that will strengthen the behavior.

There are also difficulties when using punishment as a technique to decrease behavior:

- A problem behavior must be allowed to occur

- A consequence must be chosen that is aversive enough to be effective

- The side effects of using punishment must be dealt with. Nobody likes punishment, even mild punishment like reprimands, loss of privileges, or similar methods typically used in class. Often students will react in negative ways to a teacher's attempt to punish including *escalation of the problem behavior*

While the *sole* use of consequences as a teaching technique has its strong and weak points, we see from the Behavior Change Timeline that consequences are only half the story. Antecedents also have a strong effect on behavior. In the next chapter we will focus on the potent methodology involved in manipulating antecedents to achieve a desirable behavior change.

Key Concepts

1. Why does the scientific study of behavior require that behavior be defined in observable and objective terms? What's wrong with mentalistic descriptions of behavior like, "He was happy all day."

2. State the components of the Behavioral Timeline.

3. What are contingencies?

4. Name four kinds of contingencies or consequence-based procedures.

5. Define each consequence-based procedure with respect to *operation* and *function*. Provide an example of each involving students with autism.

6. Give an example illustrating the *shaping* of a new behavior by reinforcing *successive approximations*.

7. Name some limitations of *sole* use of reinforcers and punishers.

Resources and References

See the list at the end of the next chapter.

Chapter 2

Antecedents:
Building Blocks to a Proactive Educational Environment

Behavior change techniques are *proactive* if they occur before the behavior (they are antecedents) and they have an effect on making some behaviors occur more or less often. For example, off-task behaviors may be decreased when loud noise is eliminated from an environment where reading is about to occur. Reading may be promoted by posting colorful advertisements that illustrate interesting books.

Let's take a look in summary at the main techniques of manipulating antecedent conditions in an educational setting.

Summary

1. Keep the Student Busy
Keep instruction fast paced and moving. Reinforce appropriate alternative behaviors at a high rate.

2. Stack the Deck
Choose potent and varied reinforcers and have plenty available.

3. Eliminate the Competition
Make competing reinforcers and other distractions unavailable as much as possible.

4. Structure the Physical Environment
Set up the classroom or learning area so that it propels students into learning and decreases the opportunities for off-task or misbehavior.

5. Maximize Choice and Individual Control
Build choice and preference into the curriculum. Recognize that too many rules and obvious controls can be counterproductive and provoke rebellion.

6. Ensure Readiness
Make sure that the child has the prerequisite skills for accomplishing the tasks set before them and that the requirements are not too hard.

7. Teach Errorlessly
Analyze the skill into its component parts and develop a strategy to teach it a little at a time, starting with the simplest parts and minimizing errors.

8. Allow the Student to Be Competent
Plan the daily schedule so that children are spending a significant amount of time performing things that they CAN do.

9. Know Your Enemy
Where problem behavior exists, understand WHEN and WHY it occurs.

10. Intervene Early
Problem behaviors usually start subtly and could be much more easily taken care of if we are on the alert for them

11. Listen to the Student
The behavior of the student is the most reliable indicator of how things are going. Learn to analyze it carefully and objectively.

12. Stay Calm and Have Fun
Students take their emotional cues from teachers.

Picture yourself getting ready to teach a 5-year-old with autism. You are responsible for implementing programs in a variety of subject areas and settings. The student is easily distractible, poorly motivated, and has major tantrums during structured learning time. How would you set up the teaching programs? What do you need to consider and how should you prepare? Let's discuss the building blocks and discuss how arranging antecedents can address these and other issues of program design.

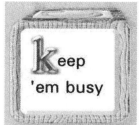

PACING

No one likes to be bored. T.V. advertisers know this and change images in their commercials so often it can be dizzying. Viewers sit on their couches with the ultimate decision making tool—the remote control—and mercilessly change the channel, seeking out programs that grab their attention. The unfortunate ones that do not produce immediate and intense gratification are gone in a click.

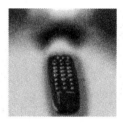

Students can be like this and vote with their attention and behavior. They "change the channel" by looking out the window, doodling in their notebooks, talking to a friend, or daydreaming. If they are uncomfortable or bored enough they may even protest or try to escape the situation. As in advertising, pacing is crucial in teaching. The teacher needs to know what should be done at every moment. The plan of instruction should always include more than enough material to keep students engaged and active.

Actually, "pacing" is comprised of several things. Keeping students connected with the material is accomplished in at least three steps:

- Engaging
- Pacing and Presentation
- Responding

Engaging means that the teacher obtains the students' attention before proceeding with instruction. Once connected, the teacher does everything possible to maintain the student's attention.

Pacing and Presentation means that after the student is engaged, the presentation of material must be as rapid as can be tolerated by the student, with no gaps, hesitation, or dead space. This really takes preparation and practice on the part of the teacher, almost like the choreography of a ballet.

When students react to the teacher's instruction, the teacher must *respond* in the appropriate way. The teacher could reinforce, punish, or redirect behavior, re-present or rephrase the instructional material, or do other things. Whatever is done should be done smoothly, without hesitation, maintaining the engagement of the student with the material.

Opportunities to Respond

Reading a story to a group of three-year-olds without pausing to ask questions or respond to comments will quickly result in a group of inattentive children. Students must have frequent opportunities to respond to the material so that reinforcement can occur often. Gauge your audience and build in frequent opportunities to respond to the material in whatever way is appropriate for them. Think of this as the "AMEN! Principle." Religious leaders giving a sermon are sometimes grateful for a congregation that responds often to the things that they say. They often phrase their remarks to elicit a lively response ("AMEN!") as often as possible because they believe that an active response from the congregation results in better retention of the message. You should do the same with your teaching.

******

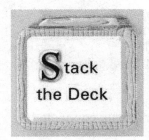

If you engage your students, hold their attention, and give them lots of opportunities to respond they will receive many reinforcers. Of course, reinforcers take different forms including praise, privileges, approval from peers, good grades, and preferred edibles. The quality of these consequences or others will go a long way towards determining the motivation level of your students. Use the most potent reinforcers you can find.

Individualize your reinforcers. Make sure the reinforcing event is motivating to a particular student. If you don't know, ask the student, experiment, or interview others.

Use novelty and plan for satiation. Understand that, sometimes, things can be reinforcing just because they are new or unexpected. Use this principle by changing aspects of reinforcing events as often as necessary. Don't just use one phrase if you're praising someone's work; use several and add new ones all the time. Change the toys, edibles, activities, or privileges that are awarded before they lose their effectiveness. Understand that, eventually, most things will lose their effectiveness so have new potential reinforcers in the wings.

You might ask how this connects with antecedents since reinforcement is a consequence to behavior. Remember that the reinforcers you use are aspects of the setting as soon as they become apparent to students. Their availability is part of the antecedent environment.

******

As a teacher you have a rival. This rival mercilessly competes with you for the attention of your students and it often wins. Your opponent is the distractions and alternative activities available to your students instead of paying attention to you or completing their work.

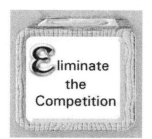

Talking with friends, doodling in notebooks, daydreaming, fidgeting, changing the subject, refusing to participate, and attempting to escape are all behaviors that can and do occur during teaching sessions. Identify specific distractions and eliminate them one by one. If a student is bothered by long sleeves (the buttons may catch on the edge of the desk) try to arrange for him to wear short sleeves. If a student looks out the window, face her away from it. Put favorite toys and irrelevant materials out of sight. Make sure students feet touch the floor, that they are relatively comfortable in their seats, and that there are no distracting noises.

Keeping students engaged in active, fast-paced instruction with many highly reinforced opportunities to respond prevents a lot of problems. Even so, sometimes instruction cannot compete with an environment full of distractions. Be alert and win the competition!

******

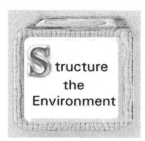

While you are arranging the environment to eliminate distractions and competing reinforcers you can also set it up to directly facilitate your instruction. Survey your instruction area and assess whether it is efficient and logical in its arrangement of materials and equipment. This is called human factors engineering (aren't you glad there's a whole specialty devoted to this?). Have you ever wondered who decides how big the buttons will be on your dashboard or where they are placed? No? Well, manufacturers are very concerned with making products that are easy to use. When materials and equipment are arranged in ways that make them easy to use, we think less about finding and using them and more about the task at hand. In your teaching situation, be your own human factors engineer and consider your environment:

- How big is the room or teaching space?
- What else is occurring at the same time as your instruction?
- How are desks, tables, and chairs placed?
- How convenient are instructional materials to the teacher who will use them?
- How large are diagrams? How clear are they?
- Should you pass out a handout or point to a large sample on the board? (Some groups play with the papers rather than pay attention).
- How long is the task? Does it exceed the tolerance of some?
- What time of day is the instruction given? What comes before and what comes after?
- How big is the group?
- What is the composition of the group, personalities, learning abilities?

Teaching is like serving a great meal. In addition to the food itself (teaching presentation), the dishes, tablecloth, lighting, and music (environmental factors) make important contributions to the overall dining (learning) experience.

******

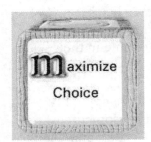

Children are not empty containers into which we deposit our teaching. They react and interact with our instruction according to their own abilities, learning styles, and preferences. Regrettably, sometimes our instruction leaves them out of the equation when we fashion a program and implement it as if the student's own goals and agenda were irritatingly irrelevant. Our attempts to motivate the student communicate that we care about whether she learns or not. Building choice and preference into instruction says the same. Choice of reinforcers to work for, topics to write about, which play activity to spend time on, or which friends to go to lunch with, helps to engage the student in the activity and prevent non-compliance.

Known preferences can be incorporated if students are not capable of directly communicating choices. Preferred items or foods serve well as reinforcers; preferred activities serve well as topics of conversation; preferred T.V. characters serve well as instructional aids ("Big Bird is going to cut a pizza into three pieces..."). Too many externally imposed rules and obvious controls are counterproductive and will provoke rebellion. This is the opposite of choice and individual control. Certainly the teacher must set the overall agenda for instruction but if no consideration is made for preference, choice and individual control, non-compliance or disengagement will soon follow.

******

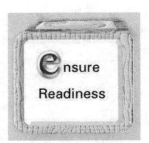

Behavior analysts have observed that a proportion of children that engage in problem behavior in classrooms do so because the tasks are too hard. Yet the same students may be initially characterized as lazy, inattentive, belligerent, non-compliant, or unmotivated. Is it the "non-compliance" or "inattentiveness" that causes the lack of acceptable work performance or the opposite—the work is hard and the child is trying to escape it?

Good teaching begins at a point where the student is competent and builds on that performance. Piano lessons start with simple pieces and progress gradually to more complicated ones. When starting a new area of instruction we need to assess the student's initial level of ability in the area. Furthermore, even once we are started we must be open to going back to earlier material if the student begins to falter.

Here are some landmarks that can alert you to problems with prerequisites:

- Is the student having problems attending even on days that they are motivated in other areas?

+ Does the student say, "I don't like (subject)"?

+ Is the student getting questions right at about the same level as chance (50% in a two-choice situation or 25% in a four-choice situation)?

+ Does problem behavior occur more just before, during, or just after the instruction in question?

Some students have truly mastered the prerequisites but just don't like things that require a lot of effort, like new tasks. This is more of a reinforcer problem than anything else. Other students could not accomplish the task no matter how motivated they are. It is important to distinguish the latter from the former.

******

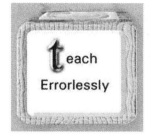

In order to know where the student must start in an instructional area you must first analyze the target skill into its component parts and develop a strategy to teach it a little at a time, starting with the simplest parts. This is called *errorless teaching* because it minimizes the chance of errors on the part of the student. Errors are not beneficial to learning. Errors mean the student is practicing and strengthening the *wrong* performance. As a wise man (Dr. Larry Stoddard of Northeastern University) once said, "Errors beget errors." If you teach a little bit at a time, building small performances on top of those just learned, you will maximize the success of the student and minimize failure.

The analysis of the skill to be learned (called a *task analysis*) is crucial to understanding what is to be taught. A partial task analysis is illustrated below for the independent living skill tooth brushing:

1. Unscrew cap from toothpaste
2. Pick up toothbrush
3. Squeeze toothpaste onto toothbrush
4. Put toothpaste down
5. Turn on water
6. Place toothbrush underneath water
7. etc. for additional steps

Of course, not all skills are simple to analyze. Expressive language includes numerous sub-skills like asking for desired objects, greeting others, naming common objects, naming verbs and actions, and naming people and places. Play, reading, addition, social interaction, and chemistry all represent complex subjects that can be task analyzed. It is this analysis that provides the foundation, sequence, and scope for instruction.

If presenting a simpler task to a student still does not result in a correct performance, errorless methodology gives the student various forms of assistance, generally called *prompts*. These prompts are antecedents that take many different forms including physical, verbal, written, or environmental forms. Prompts are designed to give the student enough help to achieve a correct performance and positive reinforcement. After the student's correct performance is strengthened prompts are gradually faded until the student is correct independently. (Additional information on task analysis, prerequisites, prompts, and the manipulation of antecedents can be found in Section II – Teaching Formats.)

******

Ask a teacher the purpose of school and you're sure to get an answer along the lines of, "For learning new things, of course!" Although not incorrect, there is more to the question than is apparent. Consider what proportion of the day is spent in various kinds of activities for students. What would you think is the most productive allocation of time for them? Should they spend most of their time trying to do things that they are learning to do (can *not* yet do independently) or should they spend most of their time doing things that they can *already* do independently? Would it be a waste of time for students to work on things that they already know how to do? Think about your own life. Imagine spending the majority of your time doing things that you are incompetent to do? Sound like fun? Picture your boss leaning over your shoulder, giving you physical guidance each step of the way while you do your job.

There is an optimal balance in any daily schedule between performing activities in which we are autonomous and competent, and working on achieving new skills. Plan your students' day to include enough time for independence so that children are spending a significant amount of time performing things that they CAN do. Competence breeds independence and responsibility.

******

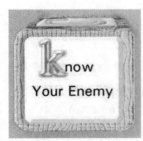

It pays to understand *why* and *when* problem behavior occurs. All behavior, including problem behavior, functions in some way for an individual. The process of figuring out how the behavior functions is called *functional analysis*. Functional analysis can be an involved process and is covered in detail elsewhere in the behavioral literature. However, without too much thought, you may already have a good idea about why and when a problem behavior occurs and, also, where, and with whom it occurs. This can help you in planning instruction. Recognize that behavior usually occurs for one or more of the following reasons:

- To obtain desired materials, activities, or privileges (toys, edibles, money, etc.)

+ For attention from others (praise, laughs, recognition, time with a favorite person)

+ To obtain pleasurable sensations intrinsic to the activity (rocking, dancing, hugging)

+ To escape or avoid an unpleasant event (difficult tasks, non-preferred activities, people or settings)

+ As a reaction to other people's attempts to compete with or control the individual's behavior

(Adapted from Iwata et al., 1990)

Just knowing these facts about what maintains a behavior suggests things that you can do to make them less likely to occur. For example, if you know that a student is misbehaving to get out of certain task requirements, you would probably do everything possible to deal with the behavior without having him leave the situation or be excused from having to do the work. With problem behaviors, knowledge is power.

******

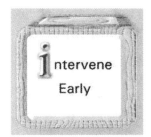

Intervene
Early

Problem behaviors usually start subtly and could be more easily taken care of if we were on the alert for them. Behavior analysts talk about a *chain* of behaviors. If you intervene *early* in the chain you can redirect behavior before it gets going.

Scientists know this principle well. Recently, considering the remote possibility that a large asteroid may one day hit the earth, destroying all life, they recommended monitoring the skies to facilitate early detection so that attempts to redirect the asteroid would be made early in it's path towards the earth. That's because early in the asteroid's course it is only necessary to deflect it a fraction of a degree in order to ensure that it will miss the earth by hundreds of thousands of miles. Later on, however, when it is closer, it will take much more force and require a much greater deflection. In teaching our worries are closer to home. But, if we can identify the beginnings of problem behavior (minor complaints, fidgeting, pauses in responding, inattention) we may be able to respond to them to get the student back on track. Our responses could take various forms. We might make the task slightly easier, give more examples, reinforce more often, stop earlier, or change to a different task altogether. In any case, it is far easier to salvage the session by making minor accommodations early than deal with a major disruption later.

******

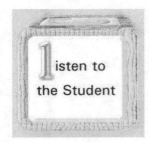

The advice "listen to the student" should be taken literally as well as figuratively. Students often tell us exactly what is going on with them, what they like, and what they don't. We need to listen to them and take what they say seriously. Value judgments about students ("lazy", "unmotivated", "immature", etc.) can sometimes be excuses for lack of teaching success and have little place in good teaching.

The behavior of the student is the most reliable indicator of how things are going. Learn to analyze it objectively and accept what it tells you about what you are doing. To paraphrase B. F. Skinner, "The student is always right." This means that the behavior of the student is always lawful and largely results from environmental influences. As a teacher you are a big part of the environment and must constantly revise and adapt your instruction to the needs and abilities of your students.

******

Most parents with little children have seen them fall and scrape a knee or arm. When the injury is slight there may be a moment when the child is silent and looks up at the parent, as if trying to decide how to react. Does this hurt? Should I cry? Is this serious? At this time the parent's tone of voice and facial expression supply the child with the answers to those questions.

Students take their emotional cues from teachers too. If students are uncomfortable or annoyed we can sometimes make it worse or better, depending on our tone of voice, facial expression, and general demeanor. A calm exterior and steady voice, no matter what is going on inside, will go a long way towards reassuring students that you are in control. It may also signal to them that their problem behavior will not be reinforced with your attention or by disrupting a situation. Even beyond dealing with problem behavior, a friendly and confident manner sets the tone for compliance and cooperation from students. It says that you are someone whom they can trust to set rules that will be fun as well as productive and educational.

Key Concepts and Questions

1. Discuss how to keep students engaged. Include the concepts of pacing and presentation, and opportunities to respond.

2. Discuss the importance of individualization, novelty, and satiation in choosing reinforcers.

3. Evaluate a particular teaching environment and discuss ways to eliminate distractions.

4. Using the same environment chosen above, discuss ways to arrange it differently so that learning is better facilitated.

5. How can choice be incorporated for students who do not directly communicate choices.

6. What is a task analysis? How is it used in errorless teaching?

7. Task analyze the skill of riding a bicycle.

8. Why are mistakes counterproductive to learning?

9. What is functional analysis?

10. Name two general reasons why behavior occurs.

11. Why intervene early with problem behaviors?

References and Resources

Cooper, J. O., Heron, T. E., & Heward, W. L. (1987). *Applied Behavior Analysis.* New York, NY: Macmillan Publishing Company, 866 Third Avenue, New York, NY 10022.

Iwata, B. A., Vollmer, T. R., & Zarcone, J. R. (1990). The experimental (functional) analysis of behavior disorders: methodology, applications, and limitations. In A. C. Repp & N. N. Singh (Eds.) *Perspectives on the use of nonaversive and aversive interventions for persons with developmental disabilities* (pp. 301-330). Sycamore, IL: Sycamore Publishing Company.

Johnston, J. M. & Pennypacker, H. S. (1993). *Strategies and Tactics of Behavioral Research (Second Edition).* Hillsdale, NJ: Lawrence Erlbaum Associates, Publishers.

Martin, G. & Pear, J. (1983) *Behavior modification: What it is and how to do it.* Englewood Cliffs, NJ: Prentiss-Hall.

Part II: Teaching Formats and Settings

Introduction

Methodologies of behavior change have two important aspects: the *techniques* or specific procedures employed and the underlying learning *principles*. For example, *positive reinforcement* is a basic learning principle, but delivering a small piece of candy contingent on the occurrence of a specific behavior is a technique. The popularization of applied behavior analysis has led to great general interest in the field but especially in the techniques used. Particular techniques have even become associated with the names of prominent practitioners (e.g., the *Lovaas* method). This is not necessarily a bad thing; original ideas and creative methodology lead to progress both in ABA research and clinical work. Without new developments the field becomes static and will, ultimately, fail to solve the complex problems that remain. However, the popularization of techniques must not occur at the expense of an understanding of the basic principles involved. For quite some time behavior analysts have resisted a "cookbook" approach to methodology—the simplistic prescription of behavior change techniques without prior analysis of factors affecting behavior in a particular case or situation. The advocacy of technique without such assessment can lead to misunderstandings and misapplications of behavior analytical technology. Good ABA programs match methodology to a clear understanding of the target skill and the student's learning style including reinforcement history, interfering behaviors, and needs for structure, novelty, and pacing.

Choice of a Teaching Format

Only individual student assessment will lead teachers towards the choice of an appropriate behavior change technique or *teaching format*. The following sections will discuss various techniques or formats used to teach a variety of skills in a variety of settings. Each has a valid place in the continuum of methodologies required in the learning lives of young children. In addition to describing the format and some techniques involved, each section will discuss underlying behavior principles, target skills, and application considerations. Together, these formats, settings, and skill areas offer a broad range of options for setting up a comprehensive educational program.

Chapter 3

TEACHING IN DISCRETE TRIALS

The term *discrete trials* refers to a series of learning opportunities with a definite beginning and end. These "trials" usually occur in a short series with a student seated at a table away from distractions. Discrete trial methodology is usually adult directed, with one teacher assigned to each student. For this reason the format can be described as individualized. Reinforcers, pacing, and target skills are all arranged specifically for the individual student. This helps to maximize the potential that the child will be engaged and learn at a fast rate. Each student usually is given a unique space in which his or her learning materials are arranged. This allows teachers to keep presentation of materials fluid and consistent. Data is immediately taken on student performance and allows accurate, frequent and detailed analysis of progress.

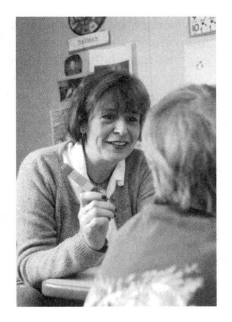

The capacity for individualization and consistent presentation of skill programs combined with the brevity and frequency of learning opportunities make discrete trials a powerful format However, some practitioners have criticized the discrete trial format as unnecessarily repetitive and not motivating, with limited spontaneous generalization to settings other than the training environment. These criticisms seem to arise from observations of student difficulties during discrete trial teaching sessions. For example, some students vehemently resist being seated for more than brief periods of time. Other forms of noncompliance and marked inattention can also be prominent during discrete trials for some students. These are often students for whom motivation and sustained attention is a severe problem in general. Unfortunately, the methodology of discrete trial teaching is not completely standardized and considerable variations in implementation exist, making it more difficult to assess the validity of the criticisms. Nevertheless, in the following chapter, the principles of teaching in discrete trials will be presented with particular attention paid to discussion of motivation and the factors that influence active participation and engagement of the student with the learning task.

Arranging Learning Opportunities in Trials

At the most fundamental level, all discrete trial procedures teach in trials. A trial begins by obtaining the student's attention and presenting an instruction of some type.

The student is then given the opportunity to respond and, if the desired response is emitted, the student is reinforced. These four basic events are illustrated in the figure below.

1. Obtain Student's Attention

The student is often seated in an area away from distractions and oriented in a manner that is comfortable and convenient. The environment is arranged to suit the activity, with materials (including data sheets) and reinforcers available. The teacher is seated in a place where the student is able to see the teacher's face and any materials used. The period of time before the trial begins is used to promote good attention on the part of the student. The teacher may engage the child in a playful manner as the child is being seated, hoping to be able to give the first instruction without ever losing the student's attention. Sometimes, when the teacher is ready to begin, it may be sufficient to simply pause and wait for the student to make eye contact. This may occur especially with highly motivated individuals, those with experience with this form of teaching, or once a series of successful trials has been initiated and the child continues to be engaged with the activity and teacher.

Four Events of a Trial

1. Obtain Student Attention
2. Present Instruction
3. Student Responds
4. Deliver Consequence

If the student does not automatically give his or her attention to the teacher at the start of the trial, the teacher may need to attract the child's attention in some way. Sometimes simply saying the child's name or "look" is sufficient. Another method is to attract the attention of the child by showing the reinforcer. When the child reaches for it the object is "swept" up near the eyes of the teacher in order to shift the gaze of the child towards the teacher's face. With some skill programs (such as object naming) the teacher shows an object to the student as part of the initial instruction (e.g., "What's this?"). Varying the position of the object shown (high, low, left, right) from trial to trial can help hold the student's interest and attention. Obtaining the student's attention with extra prompts, while necessary in some cases, should not become a permanent part of the trial. Effort should be made to fade prompts as soon as possible so that the child does not learn to wait for prompts before paying attention to the teacher.

The duration of the trial and the timing of moving from trial to trial (pacing) is important. Once the child responds correctly and a reinforcer is delivered, the child's attention should be maintained by the teacher by starting the next trial as soon as the reinforcing event is accomplished. In addition to reinforcing the target behavior of the skill program, some teachers try to increase unprompted attention to the teacher by occasionally reinforcing the student just for making eye contact and sitting correctly.

Factors that may interfere with Attending to the Teacher

Spontaneous attention to the teacher would normally be expected if the student has learned that the teacher is the source of highly desirable items, events, or interactions. Making the delivery of these stimuli contingent on the occurrence of a specific target behavior is central to discrete trial methodology. However, several factors can adversely affect the likelihood that a student will attend to the teacher.

- The reinforcer chosen by the teacher may not be desirable at a particular moment in time
- Other reinforcers in the environment may compete for the student's attention
- The difficulty or duration of the task may make some consequences insufficient to maintain responding

Each of these problems requires adaptations in teaching strategy. For example, in some cases, a choice of reinforcers might be offered to a student or the student may be asked what they would like to work for. Reinforcers could be rotated to keep them novel. However, sometimes, despite such adaptations, a student will remain unmotivated and inattentive. In such cases an incidental teaching format may be more productive (see Chapter 5).

2. Present Instruction

Most skill programs have a particular instruction that is designed to signal the student to engage in a particular target behavior (e.g., "Match", "Do this" (with model of action), "Shake bell"). These early learning tasks require the student to *discriminate*. In everyday language, learning to discriminate means to be able to tell the difference between objects, features, actions, etc. A *discriminating* wine connoisseur can tell the difference between a good and bad wine; a *discriminating* theater critic compares and contrasts films. Young children learning about the world around them need to learn to discriminate between shapes, colors, objects, noises, people, and the various forms of spoken language as well as innumerable other things. With discrete trial methodology this begins with presenting the instruction.

Most skill programs require discriminations called *conditional discriminations,* where the student learns to follow an instruction given by the teacher. The "instruction" can be a word or sentence, presentation of an object, action, or anything else that is designed to communicate to the student what to do. This instruction usually starts out having no meaning to the student but, after a number of reinforced trials, the instruction comes to control the student's behavior. Once the instruction controls the student's behavior it is properly called a *discriminative stimulus* or S^D. For example, illustrating with a matching task, on one trial a student is presented with a picture of a ball and a teacher says, "Match." In order to be correct the student must pick out (discriminate) an identical picture of a ball from among several pictures and place his picture on top. On the next trial the teacher gives the student a picture of a star and says, "Match" which requires the student to find the star and place his picture on top of that picture. The discrimination performance required of the student on both trials is dependent or *conditional* on the instruction given (picture + "Match").

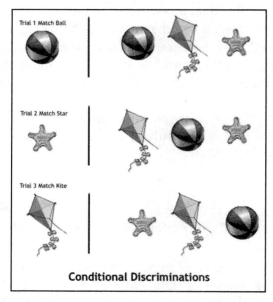

Conditional Discriminations

In identical matching, the instruction is an object or photo that exactly matches only one of the choices that are placed before the student. Other types of matching include finding items that match just some aspects of the sample like its color, shape, construction, size, position, or order. Sometimes the common aspects between a sample and a matching choice are subtle, as when similar but non-identical shoes are matched. Abstract relationships can also be taught between the sample and matching stimuli as when socks are matched to shoes (called *associations* in some curriculums), or objects are placed together according to category names (*categories*). For every task, the student uses the information contained in the initial "instruction" to complete the task. Many types of discriminations are taught in a typical early learning curriculum, such as labels (e.g., choosing a picture of a cat in response to a spoken word "cat") and following instructions but more advanced subjects like reading, mathematics, spelling, writing, and most other skills also contain discrimination performances.

3. Student Responds

Teaching personnel must have a specific, objective definition of the target behavior, which is usually contained in the written skill program. A mastery criterion is set for each target behavior that defines when it is time to move on to new performances. The *difficulty of the task* is an important concern and complex skills are usually simplified by breaking them into smaller, more easily learned component skills. Furthermore, a more successful performance can be obtained by *adapting teaching materials* and *providing helping prompts*, gradually withdrawing them as the student becomes more independent. (All of these concepts are discussed in greater detail later in this chapter.)

4. Deliver Consequence

If the student responds correctly, a potent reinforcer should be delivered immediately, together with enthusiastic praise. As discussed earlier, the potency of the reinforcer is quite important—students quickly become bored, inattentive, and even uncooperative when consequences are weak or not interesting to them. If the student makes a mistake the teacher conducts an error correction procedure (see later in this chapter).

Inter-trial Interval

The time between trials (*inter-trial interval*) should be kept as short as possible, which can be challenging to teaching personnel who must reinforce the child, mark the data sheet, remove any materials of the preceding trial and set up the materials for the next trial. Nevertheless, the momentum of success and the interest of the child are at stake and a proper flow of instruction should be maintained, avoiding delays created by extraneous movement and looking for materials.

Skill Programs

When the child is first acquiring a new skill in the discrete trials format, a series of trials is usually conducted for a single skill program in order to give the student repeated opportunities to master the desired performance. The number of trials in each session is not standard and depends on the student's learning history and the particular target behavior. If the student is highly motivated by intrinsic aspects of the task or by consequences delivered by the teacher, and the task is relatively easy, higher numbers of trials may be conducted without difficulty. However, the quality of the trial is more important than the quantity of trials. Three or four trials where the student is highly attentive, responds correctly, and receives an exciting consequence are more beneficial than 10 or more trials of weak performances, many errors, and mediocre consequences. Successful trials have a tendency to lead to more successful trials, building momentum as the series proceeds, so it is important to obtain correct responding early. When presenting more difficult steps, some teachers lead off with a few trials of a mastered performance in order to begin building momentum, and then switch to the target step. For example, if a student is having difficulty learning to match identical colors, the session may begin with a few picture matching trials that were previously mastered. After successful responses to the picture matching trials, the teacher, smoothly and without interruption, switches to the first color matching trial.

As the series of trials proceeds, the teacher must determine the appropriate place to end, based on the student's performance rather than on any arbitrarily determined point. As it is important to begin with a positive performance, it is also necessary to end with one. When the teacher gains experience with the individual student on a task, it will be easier to find the optimal ending point, balancing the need for productive practice with the risk that inattention due to fatigue or reinforcer satiation may lead to errors.

Skill programs may be conducted consecutively or with short breaks inserted depending on the history of the student and the nature of the programs. In determining the frequency and duration of breaks, once again, the most important factors are student related. While it is desirable to gradually increase the amount of time that a student can productively work, this must not be done at the expense of the student's motivation to be involved in the work. If students are given short "breaks," this time should not be viewed as a break from learning. (See the section "Creating and Maintaining a Student Schedule" in Chapter 8.)

Mixing Drills

One specific activity that will promote both maintenance of learned skills and generalization is to *mix skill programs* in the discrete trial setting. As specific skill programs are mastered they must be maintained or they will be forgotten. One way to do this is to mix them together in a teaching session where a trial or two of each drill is randomly presented to the student. This is also an excellent way of promoting the receptive language skills involved in listening carefully to instructions. A typical set of trials might look like the following. A teacher sits at a table with a child. Many objects and materials previously used in instruction are available. The teacher displays the items or points to things as necessary.

Trial	Teacher Instruction:
1	"Point to nose."
2	"Show me red."
3	"Show me green."
4	"Where's the truck?"
5	"Where's *my* hand?"
6	"Where's *your* hand?"
7	"Where's *my* hair?"
8	"Where's *your* hair?"
9	"Touch the block."
10	"Find the table."
11	"Do this." (Claps hands)
12	"Turn around."
13	"Match." (Gives object)
14	"What's this?" (Shows car)

The variety of instructions must be increased gradually and systematically but since only mastered drills are included as instructions, the main task for the student is to listen to the instruction and identify which of the performances already in his repertoire are required.

Generalization

Discrete trial teaching as well as teaching in other formats usually involves learning new skills under somewhat specific conditions. If a student learns to name objects in one setting (like an individual space free from distractions) he may not necessarily name objects during snack or at home. Each skill acquired in isolation must be specifically trained to occur *in other settings, with other people, and even when using slightly different instructions and materials*. (See the section on *Stimulus Lists* later in this chapter for a method of documenting generalization in skill programs.) It is important to avoid thinking that a skill program is completed when it is mastered in isolation. Skills must continue to be practiced until they occur in a variety of settings, with a variety of people, and in response to a variety of slightly different instructions or materials.

Designing Skill Programs

Breaking Skills into Simple Steps

It is important to appreciate the complexity of new skills as preparations are made for teaching in discrete trials. Generally, complex skills are broken down into simpler, component parts and the student is asked to learn in small steps, judging that difficult tasks are best learned a little at a time. Small steps will help to ensure that the student is reinforced often and that discouraging errors will be avoided. For example, the skill of tooth brushing can be broken down into many smaller component steps—*taking the cap off the toothpaste, picking up the toothbrush, putting paste on brush, turning on water,* etc. A student is taught these steps one at a time in order to make the learning easier and more manageable. This is called a *sequential* skill analysis. Some skills require a different kind of simplification process called a *hierarchical* skill analysis—rather than breaking up a skill into a sequence or chain of behaviors, prior mastery of other more fundamental skills is needed. For example, in order to name colors, one must be able to visually discriminate between colors. This is often taught by having the student learn to match identical colored cards or objects. In order to match cards, the student needs to be able to physically place them on top of each other. It is also often helpful for the student to identify pictures of the colors when the teacher names them ("Touch red"). Therefore, at least three performances are prerequisite to naming colors: placing cards on cards, color matching, and identifying colors named by the teacher. The diagram above illustrates the relationships. Every skill has its own list of prerequisites and a good curriculum should indicate the sequence of how skills should be acquired.

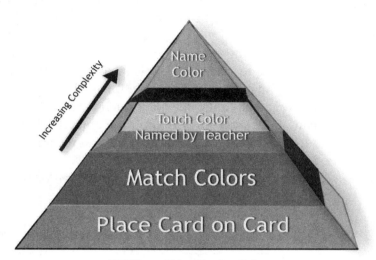

Skill Pyramid for **Naming Colors**

Arranging Teaching Materials and Stimulus Control

Teaching discriminations and other skills by breaking them into component parts and moving forward in small steps forms the basis for a more *errorless* technique of teaching. Errors interfere with learning, especially in early learning, when emerging skills are fragile. They can cause students to become unmotivated, respond less, or even abandon previously correct performances. Errorless methods of teaching are designed to ensure that the student will be correct and, therefore, reinforced. Recall the diagram of the events of a trial. Errorless methods of teaching concentrate on the second event, the delivery of the instruction. Recall that the *instruction*, broadly defined, is the way that the task is set up, the materials used, the arrangement of the room, and the prompts given. All are part of the many stimulus conditions of the task that precede the student's behavior. The student learns the task in the context of these antecedent conditions, meaning that aspects of the stimulus conditions affect their performance. Errorless teaching manipulates antecedent stimulus conditions in various ways to ensure that the student will be correct. This is called *stimulus control*.

One way of manipulating antecedent stimuli to help a student learn a task is to construct teaching materials that make a task easier to perform initially, and then gradually change the materials to achieve more difficult final performances. For example, to teach a student to write letters, they are sometimes initially given letters made of dotted lines to trace. Gradually, the dotted lines are faded or eliminated to encourage the student to write of the letters without assistance. Another example of arranging teaching materials in specific ways to facilitate learning can be given using the task of matching quantity. In this skill program, we would like the student to be able to put together cards with the same number of items. First, we make sure that the student can match pictures with multiple objects arranged in similar patterns. We start with identical objects used in both the sample and choices.

Phase 1: Matching *similar* shapes in *similar* patterns

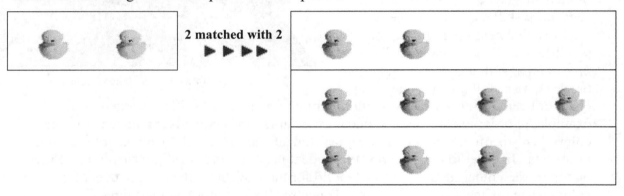

Since we want the student to pay attention to the number of items and not the shape of the items, we next teach the student to match samples to choice stimuli that are dissimilar. We could start with the following arrangement of materials:

Phase 2: Matching *dissimilar* shapes in *similar* patterns

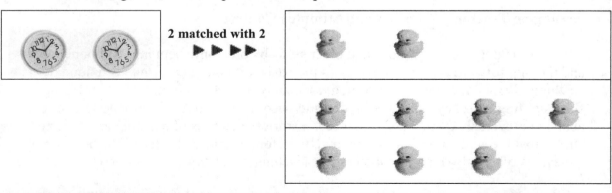

Here, the student learns to match clocks with ducks. After this is mastered we will have the student match clocks and cars, cars and ducks, dots and suns, etc. until the student is easily matching any two, three, or four objects with any other objects of the corresponding number regardless of shape. We might also gradually mix the samples and choices with different objects so that our task might end up looking like the example below:

Phase 2: Final performance

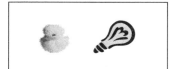

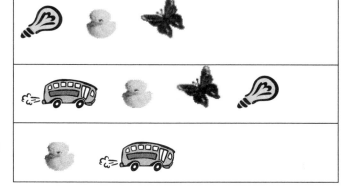

2 matched with 2
▶ ▶ ▶▶

At this point we still cannot be sure that the student is matching based on a one-to-one correspondence between the number of items in the sample and the choice. The student may be matching the pattern or arrangement of the units. In the example above, a student might learn to match on the basis of shorter groupings of objects vs. longer grouping, rather than actually look at the number of objects. If we keep the arrangement of the sample and the choice stimuli the same we cannot guarantee that the student is matching based on quantity. Therefore, for advanced students we might include an additional phase. In this phase we gradually vary the position and arrangement of the stimuli so that the student must abandon any matching strategy based on the arrangement, position, or shape of the stimuli. Initially, we move the arrangements of the stimuli very slightly and, if the student continues to respond correctly, continue the distortion of position until we arrive at the final performance as illustrated on the following page.

To summarize: in this illustration, a complex matching concept (matching quantity) is gradually taught by breaking the task into component performances. Starting with the simplest matching arrangement, the student masters tasks that successively build in complexity. Antecedent stimuli (teaching materials) are changed gradually in several dimensions (shape, position) to provide assistance to the student in maintaining a correct response while learning new steps of the task.

Phase 3: *Dissimilar* shapes in *dissimilar* patterns (final performance)

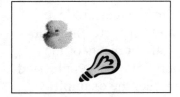

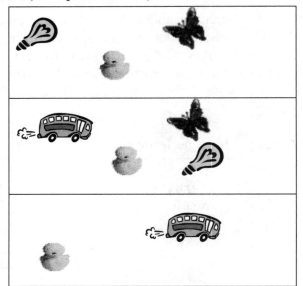

2 matched with 2
▶ ▶ ▶▶

Helping Prompts

        In addition to a gradual and systematic manipulation of the teaching materials, as
seen in the example above, a *helping prompt* of some kind may be added to the
instruction to ensure that the student will be correct. This prompt is then systematically
reduced over trials, as a way of teaching the student to respond correctly in the presence
of the instruction only. Imagine a student who is learning to imitate the gross motor
action *clap hands*. According to the program write-up, after obtaining the student's
attention, the teacher says, "Do this" and demonstrates the action. Of course, being new
to the program the student does not have the slightest idea what to do in order to be
reinforced. In errorless teaching the teacher gives the student some form of assistance
that will ensure that the student correctly engages in the target behavior and is eligible for
reinforcement. This form of assistance can be anything from physical prompts to having
another student imitate the teacher correctly; the important thing is to ensure a smooth,
errorless performance that receives reinforcement.

        Helping prompts may take the form of physical guidance and touches, written
instructions, verbal or other auditory cues, arranging the positions of items, or many other
types of prompts. Strategies of gradually eliminating the helping stimuli include
modifying the stimuli along various dimensions:

   ⊕ *Spatial*, where the position of the cue is moved and gradually located out of the
      area

   ⊕ *Temporal*, where the helping stimulus is gradually delayed more and more until
      the student anticipates the correct response,

   ⊕ *Morphological*, where the shape of the stimulus is changed, made smaller, or
      faded,

❋ *Topographical,* where the form of a movement, gesture, or touch by the teacher is gradually changed and eliminated

❋ *Auditory,* where the form of a verbal, vocal, or auditory cue is changed through pitch, volume, temporally, or another dimension.

These are called *prompt fading strategies.* For example, let's assume that the teacher chooses to physically prompt a performance. Since the objective is to have the student imitate the teacher *on his own,* some strategy must be devised to eliminate the extra help given. There are many ways that could be devised (thus, the "art" of teaching and designing curriculum) but, regardless of the fading method, we hope that at some point in fading the physical prompts the student will understand what is required for reinforcement and respond to the instruction without physical assistance.

A series of trials during prompt fading might look like the following:

Trial #	Errorless Fading Step
1	Complete hand over hand physical guidance
2	Complete hand over hand physical guidance
3	Complete hand over hand physical guidance
4	Partial hand over hand guidance
5	Partial hand over hand guidance
6	Intermittent touches
7	Intermittent touches
8	One initial touch
9	No guidance
10	No guidance
11	No guidance
12-18	No guidance

When working with a student recently, we found that he was unable to make a simple discrimination between two photos. His task was to choose the picture of a computer and not choose the picture of a clown. Unfortunately, he did not seem to be able to tell the difference between the photos. Adding a wide white border to the correct photo quickly resulted in 100% correct responding, probably because the border made the computer photo more obviously different from the clown photo. The opacity of the white border was gradually faded from 100% to 0% in 5 steps (100%, 50%, 25%, 10%, 5%) over the next 60 trials and eliminated. Although we're not sure exactly when, at some point in the fading process the student must have begun looking at the photo and not what remained of the white border.

Below is a table of examples based on a receptive language task, demonstrating how control can be shifted from several different kinds of helping prompts to the target instruction alone.

Correct Performance: Student touches photo of *Ball* when teacher says, "Ball."			
Target Instruction: Teacher says "Ball"			
Procedure: Three photos of objects on table serve as choices. Teacher says "Ball" plus:			
Point Cue Added (Temporal Fading)	**White Stripe Added (Morphological Fading)**	**Arrow Added (Spacial Fading)**	**Physical Prompts Given (Topographical Fading)**
Immediate point to correct choice	White stripe only on photo of correct choice	Correct choice has card with downward pointing black arrow positioned above it	Hand over hand guidance is used
Point to correct choice delayed by 0.5 seconds	White stripe faded to 75% opacity	Arrow is moved upwards 1 in.	Hand over hand is used but with very loose grip
Point to correct choice delayed by 1 second	White stripe faded to 50% opacity	Arrow is moved another 1 in. upwards	Continuous touch on back of hand
Point to correct choice delayed by 1.5 seconds	White stripe faded to 25% opacity	Arrow is moved another 1 in. upwards	Intermittent touch on back of hand
Point to correct choice delayed by 2 seconds	White stripe faded to 15% opacity	Arrow is moved another 1 in. upwards	Initial touch to start hand movement
Point to correct choice delayed by 3 seconds	White stripe faded to 5% opacity	Arrow is moved off table.	Motion towards hand
(Continue delay until student anticipates)	White stripe faded to 0% opacity		No prompt

For stimulus control strategies to be truly errorless a *most to least* fading strategy should be followed. This means that, initially, the maximum amount of guidance is given by the stimulus so that the student is most likely to respond correctly. As seen above the stimuli are then changed in ways that lessen their assistance gradually so that the student is prompted to shift attention from the helping stimulus to the target stimulus.

The prompts that we use to ensure an errorless performance and the strategy that we use to fade them must be matched to the student's abilities, history of reinforcement, and preferences. Furthermore, we must be sensitive from trial to trial and session to session that our strategy is working and ready to revise it when needed. Remember that the student's history and performance is, ultimately, the only important guide for implementing curriculum. Later in this chapter you will find samples of specific skill programs that include errorless procedures and stimulus control techniques.

Another example, the use of an arrow as a helping prompt, is illustrated in detail on the following page. Designing instructional materials that effectively and creatively use various kinds of prompts and prompt fading strategies is a worthwhile subject of detailed study. See the resource list at the end of this chapter for suggestions.

Example: Using and fading an arrow as a helping prompt to teach receptive identification of "Ball"

Correct Performance: Student touches photo of *Ball* when teacher says, "Ball."			
Target Stimulus: Teacher's instruction ("Ball")			
Procedure: Three photos of objects on table serve as choices. Teacher says "Ball" plus:			
Arrow Added			
Correct choice has card with downward pointing black arrow positioned above it **"Ball"**	▼ ⚽	🦁	📚
Arrow is moved upwards 1 in. **"Ball"**	🦁	▼ ⚽	📚
Arrow is moved another 1 in. upwards **"Ball"**	▼ ⚽	📚	🦁
Arrow is moved another 1 in. upwards **"Ball**	📚	🦁	▼ ⚽
Arrow is moved off table. **"Ball"**	⚽	📚	🦁

Free Responding

After prompts are faded and a student is allowed to make a response without any help from the teacher, the condition may be called *free responding*. The student is presented with the materials and given the opportunity to make a correct response, an incorrect response, or no response. If the student makes an incorrect response or does not respond, an *error correction procedure* is employed in order to attempt to help the student respond correctly in the future. Error correction can be as simple as withholding reinforcement and moving to the next trial or it can involve interrupting the incorrect action, resetting the materials, and physically prompting the student through the correct action. The choice of procedures is determined in part by the target performance, the circumstances of the error, and the materials used. Above all, reinforcement must be withheld when the correct performance is not obtained.

Sample Error Correction for Incorrect Response

1.   Smoothly interrupt incorrect action as soon as possible

2.   Return student to "ready" position, remove materials (if applicable)

3.   Do not reinforce, wait 3 seconds, no eye contact

4.   Replace stimuli in original position (if applicable)

5.   Repeat trial. Give instruction again and return to full prompts to achieve errorless performance for 1 trial

6.   Repeat trial a second time allowing unprompted choice

7.   Correct again if necessary. If a third trial in a row contains an error, return to errorless prompting condition for this performance.

Regarding step 7: sometimes an error correction procedure is not sufficient to reestablish a correct performance. When faced with an prolonged unstable performance it may be best to return to an earlier step and begin again to reestablish the problem stimulus with complete prompts before slowly fading again, rather than risk the destructive effect of more errors. Teaching is often like this—prompts may be faded as the student does well but if the student falters, prompts need to be reinstated for a time.

Conducting Skill Programs in Discrete Trials

In a typical errorless discrete trial teaching procedure all of the concepts discussed to this point are employed:

- Teaching in short, structured learning opportunities with a definite beginning and end
- Breaking skills into simple steps
- Constructing and manipulating teaching materials to enhance learning
- Adding and fading helping prompts
- Using error correction procedures with free responding

Let's illustrate such a procedure using the discrimination task of identical object matching. In this task the final target performance is to place sample objects with identical objects that are placed in a 3-object array (one correct and two incorrect choices). A student is asked to learn to match dozens of objects in this manner but must start very simply. As a first step, matching only one sample object to an identical object in a field of three choices might be required. As a helping stimulus, physical prompting is often chosen and is relatively easy to fade. Look at the table on the following page. In trials 1 – 32 we helped the student to match a sample object of *ball*, gradually fading the assistance until the student was correct on a number of consecutive trials. Once the student was independently placing the sample object with the correct choice object we again used an errorless prompting technique to teach a *second* matching performance but we also gave the student an opportunity to continue to match the first sample. When we asked for the student to match the *first* mastered stimulus, we allowed the student to respond without prompts (free responding) but when we asked for the second matching performance we prompted errorlessly.

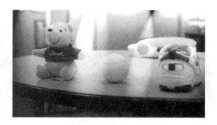

In trial 33 we began to teach the student to match a second sample (*shoe*) while maintaining the matching performance previously learned (*ball*). Physical prompts were used to achieve an errorless performance with *shoe* and faded as the trials continued, while the student was allowed to make an unprompted choice with *ball*. Since the student was allowed to make an unprompted choice with *ball* it was possible that the choice may have been incorrect, which did occur in trial 37. In this case an *error correction procedure* was implemented. In the following trial complete physical guidance was used to help the student make a correct choice on the previously incorrect stimulus. Then, the trial was repeated allowing free responding.

A General Procedure

Suggesting a general method of teaching discriminations in discrete trials is, ultimately, far too simplistic. Breaking up skills into components, selection of prompts and prompt fading strategies, and many other programming tasks must be adapted to the individual and the task at hand. There is a large body of research concerning each aspect of the teaching task that must be understood and offers guidance for many issues that are encountered with students. Such research could not be fully integrated into a simple implementation strategy. Furthermore, there are many variations of strategies that can be used, each differing in their various strengths and weaknesses and appropriate for various circumstances. However, some guidance in the form of a core procedure may be helpful to illustrate the basic procedures and can be employed as a starting point. Nevertheless, the practitioner must understand that individualized programs are essential to success and methodology must suit the student.

Table: Adding a new performance using errorless procedures while maintaining the old performance using free responding

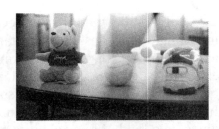

Trial #	Stimulus to Match (Correct)	Actual Student Performance	Prompts for Ball	
1	Ball	+	Complete hand over hand physical guidance	
2	Ball	+	Complete hand over hand physical guidance	
3	Ball	+	Complete hand over hand physical guidance	
4	Ball	+	Partial hand over hand guidance	
5	Ball	+	Partial hand over hand guidance	
6	Ball	+	Intermittent touches	
7	Ball	+	Intermittent touches	
8	Ball	+	Intermittent touches	
9	Ball	+	One initial touch	
10	Ball	+	One initial touch	
11-21	Ball	+	One initial touch	
22-32	Ball	+	No guidance	
Add a new performance			**Prompts for Ball**	**Prompts for Shoe**
33	Shoe	+		Complete hand over hand
34	Ball	+	No guidance (free responding)	
35	Shoe	+		Complete hand over hand
36	Shoe	+		Complete hand over hand
37	Ball	incorrect	No guidance/error correction	
38	Ball	+	Complete hand over hand	
39	Ball	+	No guidance	
40	Shoe	+		Partial hand over hand guidance
41	Shoe	+		Intermittent touches
42	Ball	+	No guidance	
43	Shoe	+		Intermittent touches
44	Ball	+	No guidance	
45	Shoe	+		One initial touch
46	Shoe	+		One initial touch
47	Ball	+	No guidance	
48	Shoe	+		No guidance
49	Shoe	+		No guidance
50	Ball	+	No guidance	
51	Shoe	+		No guidance
52	Ball	+	No guidance	
53	Ball	+	No guidance	
54	Shoe	+		No guidance

A few basic terms and methodological guidelines should be discussed at the outset. When presenting a group of materials to a student from which he or she will choose or match, present at least three objects, cards, etc. equidistant from each other and the student. This reduces the chance that students will guess correctly. From trial to trial the position of the stimuli should be randomly changed, preferably out of sight of the student. Otherwise, the student might base their performance on remembering the position or presentation order of the stimuli, rather than paying attention to the instruction. For a completely new skill program teach the first performance using errorless teaching prompts until it is exhibited independently. Then, teach a *conditional* discrimination by adding additional performances, one at a time rotating the performance required randomly. *Random rotation* occurs when several mastered performances are practiced together allowing free responding and the teacher rotates the performance required in a way that is unpredictable to the student. Again, the unpredictability of presentation is an essential ingredient of random rotation. When a new performance is first practiced with other performances using an errorless procedure, while the older performances are practiced allowing free responding, this mixed procedure is called here r*andom rotation with prompts.*

The table below presents the outline of a suggested teaching procedure. The three steps (first performance, random rotation with prompts, and random rotation) are described with suggested mastery criteria. After the first performance is mastered, steps 2 and 3 are repeated to add additional performances.

A DISCRETE TRIALS TEACHING PROCEDURE		
Step 1	**Train first performance** using errorless prompts	until an independent performance is achieved **10 times in a row**
Step 2 Random Rotation with Prompts	**Add a new performance. Practice all performances together**. Allow free responding for the old performance(s) (allow the student to choose unprompted and use a correction procedure for an incorrect performance). Use errorless prompts as needed for the new performance	until the **new** performance is obtained independently **3 times in a row** and the old performance(s) has remained 90% correct.
Step 3 Random Rotation	**Practice both performances allowing free responding** (plus error correction)	until a performance is obtained at least **80% correct** of all trials **over 2 sessions.**
Next	**Repeat steps 2-3** to add new performances	

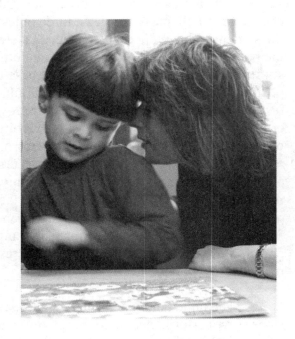

Organizing Skill Programs

Several kinds of written materials help to organize the process of teaching. *Skill programs* provide specific step-by-step instructions for conducting a given drill. Examples follow in this chapter. Other materials include *stimulus lists, data sheets,* and *graphs.* Together with other program elements discussed later under program organization, these materials help give structure to the overall program, document programming efforts, and, in general, provide a basis for evaluating quality of implementation and student progress.

Stimulus Lists

Stimulus lists provide a way of keeping track of what is being worked on in a program. They contain critical information such as the dates of implementation and mastery of each stimulus item, list items in initial acquisition and those being practiced in random rotation, and provide a central place to keep track of generalization for each skill program. Each time a program is begun, a corresponding stimulus list is placed in the main program book opposite the data sheet. Refer to stimulus lists to determine what stimuli to present and what step of a program to conduct. Assuming that by reading the skill program you know how to conduct the drill, you should have all the additional information you need on the stimulus list.

Working with Stimulus Lists

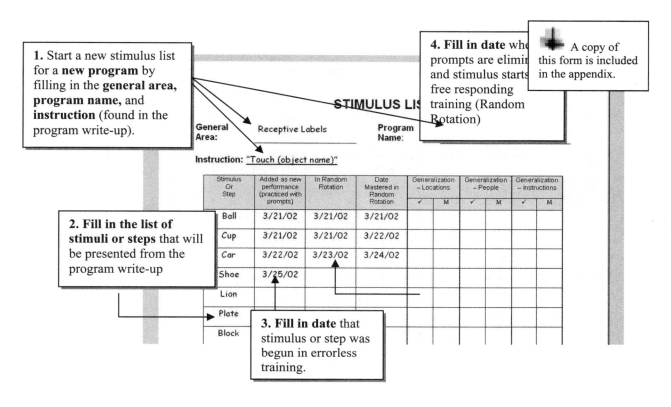

1. Start a new stimulus list for a **new program** by filling in the **general area, program name,** and **instruction** (found in the program write-up).

4. Fill in date when prompts are elimi... and stimulus starts free responding training (Random Rotation)

A copy of this form is included in the appendix.

2. Fill in the list of stimuli or steps that will be presented from the program write-up

3. Fill in date that stimulus or step was begun in errorless training.

STIMULUS LIST

General Area: Receptive Labels **Program Name:**

Instruction: "Touch (object name)"

Stimulus Or Step	Added as new performance (practiced with prompts)	In Random Rotation	Date Mastered in Random Rotation	Generalization – Locations		Generalization – People		Generalization – Instructions	
				✓	M	✓	M	✓	M
Ball	3/21/02	3/21/02	3/21/02						
Cup	3/21/02	3/21/02	3/22/02						
Car	3/22/02	3/23/02	3/24/02						
Shoe	3/25/02								
Lion									
Plate									
Block									

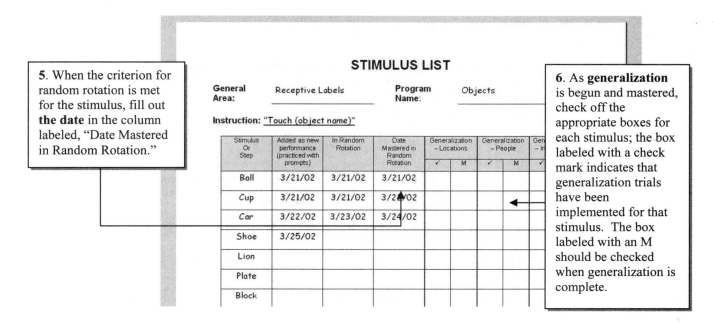

5. When the criterion for random rotation is met for the stimulus, fill out **the date** in the column labeled, "Date Mastered in Random Rotation."

6. As **generalization** is begun and mastered, check off the appropriate boxes for each stimulus; the box labeled with a check mark indicates that generalization trials have been implemented for that stimulus. The box labeled with an M should be checked when generalization is complete.

STIMULUS LIST

General Area: Receptive Labels **Program Name:** Objects

Instruction: "Touch (object name)"

Stimulus Or Step	Added as new performance (practiced with prompts)	In Random Rotation	Date Mastered in Random Rotation	Generalization – Locations		Generalization – People		Gen – I
				✓	M	✓	M	
Ball	3/21/02	3/21/02	3/21/02					
Cup	3/21/02	3/21/02	3/22/02					
Car	3/22/02	3/23/02	3/24/02					
Shoe	3/25/02							
Lion								
Plate								
Block								

Filling Out a Data Sheet

Data collection and analysis is the principle means of evaluating the effectiveness of teaching. In discrete trial teaching the results of each trial are recorded *immediately* after the trial, during the inter-trial interval.

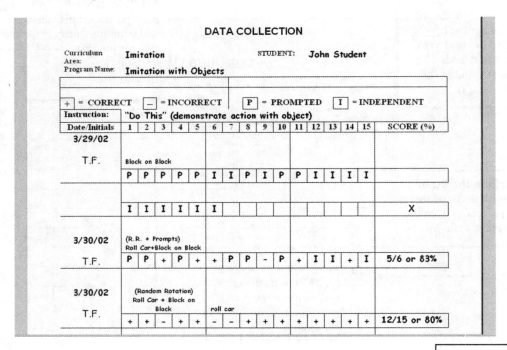

DATA COLLECTION

Curriculum Area: **Imitation**   STUDENT: **John Student**
Program Name: **Imitation with Objects**

+ = CORRECT   − = INCORRECT   P = PROMPTED   I = INDEPENDENT
Instruction: "Do This" (demonstrate action with object)

Date/Initials	1	2	3	4	5	6	7	8	9	10	11	12	13	14	15	SCORE (%)
3/29/02 T.F. Block on Block	P	P	P	P	P	I	I	P	I	P	P	I	I	I	I	
	I	I	I	I	I	I										X
3/30/02 T.F. (R.R. + Prompts) Roll Car+Block on Block	P	P	+	P	+	+	P	P	−	P	+	I	I	+	I	5/6 or 83%
3/30/02 T.F. (Random Rotation) Roll Car + Block on Block roll car	+	+	−	+	+	−	−	+	+	+	+	+	+	+	+	12/15 or 80%

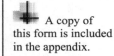 A copy of this form is included in the appendix.

1. Fill in the curriculum area, the name of the drill, the student's name, and the instruction given to start a trial.

2. Fill in the date and your initials.

3. Write down a label for the step that you are presenting to the student above the trials where you will begin recording data. Write the new stimulus name, step number, or anything that connects the data with the stimulus list.

4. Follow the code for scoring the results of each trial:

    a. During errorless teaching score (P) for prompted and (I) for independent.

    b. During random rotation with prompts score (+) for correct and (-) for incorrect for the stimuli in free responding and score (P) and (I) for the stimulus receiving prompts.

    c. During random rotation score (+) and (-) for all stimuli.

5. Start a new line for each new series of trials (but you may continue a series on the next line if more than 15 trials are given to the student).

6. During random rotation with prompts only calculate the score for stimuli not receiving prompts (free responding).

7. Calculate the score for each set of random rotation trials (percent correct). Don't calculate a percent correct unless there are at least 5 trials.

8. If a particular stimulus is incorrect two times in a row, write the name of the stimulus in the space above the incorrect marks.

Displaying Data on a Graph

Once a number of trials of data are collected a representation of that data is plotted on a graph similar to the sheet at the right. Note that there are lines evenly spaced vertically and horizontally forming a grid. The leftmost vertical line is called the *y-axis* and the bottom line that runs horizontally is called the *x-axis*.

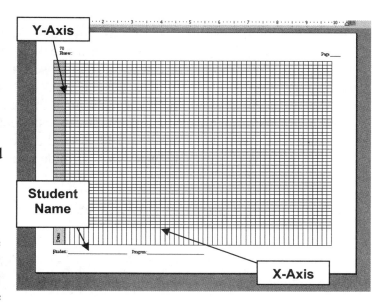

Boxes are found at the bottom of the graph where the date of each data point goes and blank spaces are located for the student's name, the program name, and page number.

As discussed in the previous section, for most programs, percent correct is graphed for a group of trials. This is accomplished in the following way:

1. Divide the number of correct trials by the total number of trials in the group.
2. Multiply the result by 100.

The resulting figure (percent of correct trials for a group of trials) is plotted on the graph. Note that there are bold horizontal lines that stretch *across* the paper. These lines begin at the X-axis and are placed every ten lines moving up the paper. Label the x-axis 0 in the gray area to the left of the line. Then label each succeeding line by adding ten, i.e., 10, 20, 30, 40, etc. up to 100. These numbers represent the percent correct. Write the label "percent correct" in the white space to the left of the y-axis.

The vertical lines represent each group of trials, one line for each group. Place your finger on the *intersection* of the zero line and the first line to the right of the Y-axis. Follow this line up until you come to a line that is close to percent correct for your group of trials. Notice that there are lines in between the bold, horizontal lines. These represent increments of 2. Use these lines to more closely approximate the place where your data should go. When you come to the intersection of the first vertical line and the horizontal line that is the closest to your percent correct, place a heavy dot. Congratulations, you've just plotted your first data point. Continue in this manner for every series of trials for this particular program. Then connect the dots with straight lines, using a ruler. Make graphs for all other programs, one graph to a program.

TOWARDS MASTERING THE CURRICULUM

Although there are hundreds of individual skills that should be learned in the early childhood curriculum, many skills fall into one of several basic areas. Since programming methodology tends to be consistent for many discrete trial programs within these areas, a sample write-up is offered here for several skills with some comments and explanations. Beginning teachers should review each sample drill carefully and be able to confidently demonstrate how each drill is performed with a student. Several published curricula are available, each with its own format and methodology but basic procedures and approach do not tend to vary greatly between the curricula. See the resource list at the end of this chapter for a list.

Sample Early Learning Programs

- **Matching**—where the student learns to put together related items
- **Gross Motor Imitation**--where the student learns to imitate actions
- **Receptive Labels**--where the student learns to identify objects when given a spoken name
- **Expressive Labels**--where the student learns to name objects
- **Receptive Instructions**--where the student learns to follow spoken instructions involving actions or objects

Sample Skill Program 1 – Identical Matching (Picture to Picture)

(You'll need two identical photos of each object for this drill. Read the skill program carefully and follow the instructions below with another person pretending to be a student.)

Stimulus List
Photos of ball, shoe, computer, cup

Matching – Pictures of Objects	
Step 1	Teacher puts three photo cards on table in front of student. Teacher obtains student's attention and says, "Match" while holding out an identical card. Using physical guidance in a *most-to-least* strategy, teacher prompts student to place the card handed to him on top of the identical card resting on the table and delivers reinforcer. Over a series of trials, as the student begins to take over the correct actions, the physical prompts are reduced and finally eliminated. The criterion for this step is reached when the student performs the correct action independently in response to the teacher's instruction 10 times in a row. (continued on next page)

Step 2 (Random Rotation with prompts)	In randomly presented trials, the teacher gives the student the photo of the *ball* or *shoe* (instruction is "Match"). For *ball* the teacher waits for a correct response (free responding). For *shoe* the teacher uses physical prompts to ensure a correct performance and fades the prompts as the student progresses. The error correction procedure is followed if errors occur on *ball*. Criterion for this step is reached when *shoe* is independently performed 3 times in a row while *ball* has been correct on at least 90% of the last 10 trials.
Step 3 (Random Rotation of both performances)	Both *ball* and *shoe* are randomly rotated and the teacher waits for a correct response. The error correction procedure is followed for incorrect responses. The criterion for this step is reached when the student performs the correct action independently in response to the teacher's instruction at least 80% of trials over two sessions for both performances.
Next	Repeat steps 2-3 for *computer* and all other new performances.

Error Correction Procedure

Calmly interrupt the student's incorrect actions as soon as possible and return the student to a ready position. The sample and choice photos are removed and the teacher waits quietly for about 3 seconds without making eye contact. Then, the choices are replaced on the table, the same instruction is again delivered and the teacher gives physical prompts to help the student perform correctly. The teacher may praise the student but withholds other reinforcement at this point. Next, when the child is ready for another trial, the teacher presents the same sample, this time giving no physical guidance. If, the student makes three errors in a row, the performance is returned to errorless prompting again.

Coaching Checklist – Step by Step

Getting Ready

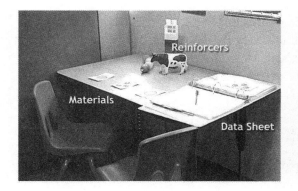
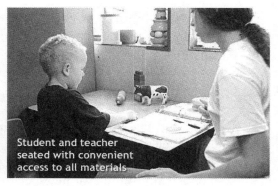

Make sure that everything is prepared before you start. It is important to avoid unnecessary interruptions.

The First Trial

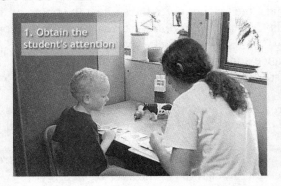 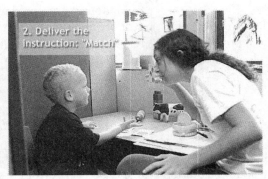

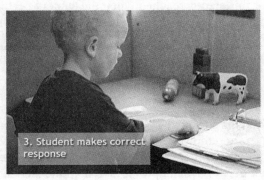 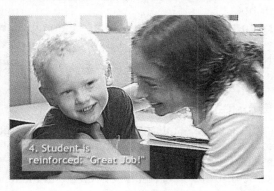

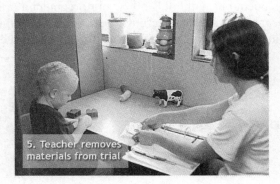 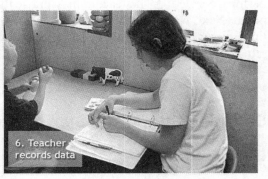

Next, get the reinforcers and materials ready for the next trial. Do a series of trials fading physical guidance until the student performs the match correctly 10 times in a row. Re-institute physical prompts as necessary

Add a new performance

1. Randomly rotate the new performance (with prompts) in trials with the old performance
2. Allow unprompted choice for old performance – use error correction if necessary
3. Use physical prompts for new performance
4. Fade physical prompts until new performance is independently achieved 3 times in a row and old performance is maintained 90% correct.
5. Practice all performances, free responding, in random rotation. Use error correction if necessary.

Sample Skill Program 2 – Imitation of Gross Motor Actions

[The basic procedure is the same as in the matching drill. The teacher's instruction ("Do this" with a model of the desired action) is the same for most imitation drills.]

Stimulus List:
Clap, pat tummy, pat head, wave

Imitation – Gross Motor Actions	
Step 1	Teacher obtains student's attention and says, "Do this" while demonstrating clapping motion. Using physical guidance in a *most-to-least* strategy, teacher prompts student to perform action and delivers reinforcer. Over a series of trials as the student begins to take over the correct actions, the prompts are reduced and finally eliminated. The criterion for this step is reached when the student performs the correct action independently in response to the teacher's instruction 10 times in a row.
Step 2 (Random Rotation with prompts for new performance)	In randomly presented trials, the teacher asks for *clap* and *pat tummy* (instruction is "Do this" with a model of action). For *clap* the teacher waits for a correct response (free responding). The error correction procedure is followed if errors occur. For *pat tummy* the teacher uses physical prompts to ensure a correct performance and fades the prompts as the student progresses. Criterion for this step is reached when the *pat tummy* is independently performed 3 times in a row while *clap hands* has been correct on at least 90% of the last 10 trials.
Step 3 (Random Rotation of both performances)	Both *clap* and *pat tummy* are randomly rotated and the teacher waits for a correct response. The error correction procedure is followed for incorrect responses. The criterion for this step is reached when the student performs the correct action independently in response to the teacher's instruction at least 80% of trials over two sessions for both performances.
Next	Repeat steps 2-3 for *pat head* and all other new performances.

Error Correction Procedure

Calmly interrupt the student's incorrect actions as soon as possible and return the student to a ready position. The teacher waits quietly for about 3 seconds without making eye contact. Then, after obtaining the student's attention, the same instruction is again delivered and the teacher gives physical prompts to help the student perform correctly. The teacher may mildly praise the student but withholds other reinforcement at this point. Next, when the child is ready for another trial, the teacher presents the same instruction, this time giving no physical guidance. Repeat error correction as needed but if the student makes three errors in a row, the performance is returned to errorless prompting again.

Sample Skill Program 3 – Receptive Labels

[Probably the most challenging part of this drill is manipulating all of the objects quickly and fluidly. Keep unused objects on a shelf or table close to you but out of sight   Remember that some objects roll and tend to fall over. This may make consistent presentation difficult.]

Stimulus List:
(3-D Objects): Truck, Barney, Ball, Cup, Spoon

Receptive Labels – 3D Objects	
Step 1	Student puts three objects on table in front of student. Teacher obtains student's attention and says, "Touch (object)" Using physical guidance in a *most-to-least* strategy, teacher prompts student to touch the object named and delivers reinforcer. After each trial the position of the three choice objects is rotated in an unpredictable way. Over a series of trials as the student begins to take over making the correct choice, the physical prompts are reduced and finally eliminated. The criterion for this step is reached when the student performs the correct action independently in response to the teacher's instruction 10 times in a row.
Step 2 (Random Rotation with prompts for new performance)	The teacher continues to rotate the position of all the choices after each trial. In random order, the teacher asks the student to touch the previously practiced object(s) and a new object. For old object(s) the teacher allows an unprompted response. An error correction procedure is followed if errors occur. For the new object the teacher uses physical prompts to ensure a correct performance and fades the prompts as the student progresses. Criterion for this step is reached when the new object is correctly chosen 3 times in a row while old object(s) has been correctly chosen on at least 90% of the last 10 trials.
Step 3 (Random Rotation of both performances)	All objects are asked for on a random basis and the teacher waits for a correct response. The error correction procedure is followed for incorrect responses. The criterion for this step is reached when the student performs the correct action independently in response to the teacher's instruction at least 80% of trials over two sessions for both performances.
Next	Repeat steps 2-3 for each new object on the stimulus list.

Error Correction Procedure

Calmly interrupt the student's incorrect actions as soon as possible and return the student to a ready position. The objects are removed and the teacher waits quietly for about 3 seconds without making eye contact. Then, the choices are replaced on the table, the same instruction is again delivered and the teacher gives physical prompts to help the student perform correctly. The teacher may praise the student but withholds other reinforcement at this point. Next, when the child is ready for another trial, the teacher presents the same instruction, this time giving no physical guidance. Repeat error correction as needed but if the student makes three errors in a row, the performance is returned to errorless prompting again

Sample Skill Program 4 – Expressive Labeling

Stimulus List (3-D Objects):
Truck, Barney, Ball, Fish (cracker)
(These items should be already mastered in Receptive Labeling.) It is necessary for the student to be able to recognizably echo the teacher's pronunciation of all words taught. This drill uses and fades verbal model prompts in the following manner:

Step	Teacher Instruction	Teacher Prompting Step	Correct Student Response
Step 1	"What's this?"	(no wait) "Truck"	"Truck"
Step 2	"What's this?"	(no wait) "Tr"	"Truck"
Step 3	"What's this?"	(no wait) "T"	"Truck"
Step 4	"What's this?"	(wait 1 sec) "T"	"Truck"
Step 5	"What's this?"	(wait 2 sec) "T"	"Truck"
Step 6	"What's this?"	(wait 3 sec) "T"	"Truck"

Expressive Labeling –Objects

Step 1	Teacher obtains student's attention and holds object in front of student. Then says, "What's this?" Using verbal modeling prompts in a *most-to-least* strategy (see above), teacher prompts student to name the object and delivers reinforcer. Over a series of trials as the student begins to readily imitate the teacher's verbal model, the prompts are faded and finally eliminated. The criterion for this step is reached when the student performs the correct action (names the object) independently in response to the teacher's instruction 10 times in a row.
Step 2 (Random Rotation with prompts for new performance)	In randomly presented trials, the teacher holds up the *truck or Barney*. For *truck* the teacher waits for a correct response. An error correction procedure is followed if errors occur. For *Barney* the teacher uses verbal modeling prompts to ensure a correct performance and fades the prompts as the student progresses Criterion for this step is reached when *Barney* is independently named 3 times in a row while *truck* has been correct on at least 90% of the last 10 trials.
Step 3 (Random Rotation of both performances)	Both *truck* and *Barney* are randomly rotated and the teacher waits for a correct response. The error correction procedure is followed for incorrect responses. The criterion for this step is reached when the student performs the correct action independently in response to the teacher's instruction at least 80% of trials over two sessions for both performances.
Next	Repeat steps 6-9 for *fish* and all other new performances.

Error Correction Procedure

The teacher looks away waits quietly for about 3 seconds. Then, after obtaining the student's attention, the object is shown and the same instruction is again delivered. At this time the teacher gives the full verbal prompt to help the student perform correctly. The teacher may praise the student but withholds other reinforcement at this point. Next, when the child is ready for another trial, the teacher presents the same instruction, this time giving no verbal prompt. Repeat error correction as needed but if the student makes three errors in a row, the performance is returned to errorless prompting again.

Sample Skill Program 5 – Receptive Instructions (Verbs)

This procedure teaches the actions associated with 10 different verbs using a single object first to help the student isolate the meaning of the verb from any particular object. By teaching the same set of verbs with additional objects, the student learns to perform the actions with any object that happens to be present. Finally, the student is taught to perform the actions with a particular object. This drill is an example of a slightly more advanced skill.

Stimulus List:
Give me, tap, shake, blow, roll, turn, drop, point to, touch, hug

Part 1: Teach stimulus list of verbs with a single object.

Receptive Instructions – Verbs with Objects	
Step 1	Teacher places a single object in center of table where student can easily reach it. Teacher obtains student's attention and gives instruction using a verb from the stimulus list, "(Verb 1)." *Teacher does not name object.* Using physical guidance in a *most-to-least* strategy, teacher prompts student to perform action and delivers reinforcer. Over a series of trials as the student begins to take over the correct actions, the prompts are reduced and finally eliminated. The criterion for this step is reached when the student performs the correct action independently in response to the teacher's instruction 10 times in a row.
Step 2 (Random Rotation with prompts for new performance)	In randomly presented trials, the teacher gives instructions using previously practiced verb(s) and a new verb. For old verbs the teacher allows an unprompted response. An error correction procedure is followed if errors occur. For the new verb the teacher uses physical prompts to ensure a correct performance and fades the prompts as the student progresses. Criterion for this step is reached when the new verb is independently performed 3 times in a row while old verb(s) has been correct on at least 90% of the last 10 trials.
Step 3 (Random Rotation of both performances)	All verbs are randomly rotated and the teacher waits for a correct response. The error correction procedure is followed for incorrect responses. The criterion for this step is reached when the student performs the correct action independently in response to the teacher's instruction at least 80% of trials over two sessions for both performances.
Next	Repeat steps 2-3 for each new verb on the stimulus list.

Part 2: Place two objects on the table and give the verb instruction including the name of one of the objects (objects should be taken from mastered list of *receptive naming.*) as in "Shake car." Follow this with the *same verb* for the second object ("Shake ball"). Randomly rotate between the two objects until the student follows the two instructions correctly. Then add a verb, randomly rotating between verbs and objects (shake ball,

shake car, tap ball, tap car). Continue adding verbs until all 10 verbs are performed randomly with both objects.

Part 3: Place another pair of familiar objects on the table and follow the procedure in Part 2. Continue in the same manner until all of the verbs are taught in combination with all of the objects or until the student begins to spontaneously follow novel combinations of verbs and objects.

Error Correction Procedure

Calmly interrupt the student's incorrect actions as soon as possible and return the student to a ready position. The teacher waits quietly for about 3 seconds without making eye contact. Then, after obtaining the student's attention, the same instruction is again delivered and the teacher gives physical prompts to help the student perform correctly. The teacher may praise the student but withholds other reinforcement at this point. Next, when the child is ready for another trial, the teacher presents the same instruction, this time giving no physical guidance. Repeat error correction as needed but if the student makes three errors in a row, the performance is returned to errorless prompting again.

Evaluating Teacher Technique

In the appendix you will find a form called the "Teaching Evaluation Checklist" that will help new teachers make sure that they are correctly performing the basic procedures of discrete trial instruction. The form is divided into several major sections:

- Structure/Setup/Environmental
- Skill Acquisition Programs
- Reinforcement/Motivation System
- Behavior Reduction Programs
- Incidental Teaching

The first 4 sections concern teaching in discrete trials. Review the form carefully before proceeding and make sure that all items are completely understood. Then, using the sample programs in the appendix, work through the programs including reinforcement, stimulus lists, and data collection with an experienced person observing and using the form to give feedback. Once you feel that you are becoming accustomed to the procedures, find a student who has already mastered the sample programs and practice the programs again. Work on fluid presentation, continuously engaging the student, and effectively reinforcing correct performance.

Summary

Discrete trial methodology is a powerful collection of procedures that provides a basic teaching approach for many children who are just beginning the curriculum and need the benefits of an intensive, highly structured format of teaching. Discrete trials is also an excellent format for intermediate and more advanced students who still require an individualized, structured approach for acquisition of new skills. The format provides a well-defined learning experience for the student with individualized target skills, presentation, pacing, and reinforcement. Specific procedures to encourage generalization of skills from the isolated environment of acquisition to a more natural setting, is an important requirement of every discrete trial program. The skill of the teacher, too, is crucial for optimal learning; time and training should be devoted to perfecting the drill presentation skills of new teachers.

Key Concepts and Questions

1. What does the word "discrete" mean in the context of this chapter?
2. What are some pros and cons to the format of discrete trials?
3. Name the four events of a trial.
4. Name the prerequisites to naming colors that were listed. Why is it important to teach skills in simpler steps?

5. What is a discrimination?

6. What is meant by "errorless teaching?"

7. How can teaching materials be arranged to facilitate learning?

8. What is a helping prompt? Name some types of prompts that could be used as a helping prompt.

9. For each prompt you named above, describe a fading strategy.

10. What is free responding?

11. Describe how errorless learning and free responding are combined to teach new performances in the general discrete trials procedure.

12. List the steps of the general error correction procedure described in the text.

13. Describe how to use the stimulus list form.

14. Describe how to use the data collection form

15. Describe how to graph data.

16. Why is generalization important? Name three kinds of generalization mentioned. Identify where to document generalization on the stimulus list form.

References and Resources

Cooper, J. O., Heron, T. E., & Heward, W. L. (1987). *Applied Behavior Analysis.* New York, NY: Macmillan Publishing Company, 866 Third Avenue, New York, NY 10022.

Holland, J. G., Solomon, C., Doran, J. & Frezza, D. A. (1976). *The Analysis of Behavior in Planning Instruction.* Reading, MA: Addison-Wesley Publishing Company,

Leaf, R. & McEachin, J. (1999). *A Work in Progress.* New York, NY: DRL Books (800) 853-1057; www.drlbooks.com

Lovaas, O. I., Ackerman, A., Alexander, D., Firestone, P., Perkins, M., Young, D. B., Carr, E. G., & Newsome, C. (1981) *Teaching developmentally disabled children: The ME book.* Austin, TX: Pro-ed; (800) 897-3202; www.proedinc.com

Martin, G. & Pear, J. (1983) *Behavior modification: What it is and how to do it.* Englewood Cliffs, NJ: Prentiss-Hall.

Maurice, C., Green, G., & Luce, S. C. (Eds.) (1996). *Behavior Intervention for Young Children with Autism.* Austin, TX: Pro-ed (800) 897-3202; www.proedinc.com

Sidman, M., & Stoddard, L. T., (1966). Programming perception and learning for retarded children. In N. R. Ellis (Ed.), *International review of research in mental retardation.* New York: Academic Press.

Terrace, H. S. (1963a). Discrimination learning with and without "errors." *Journal of the Experimental Analysis of Behavior, 6,* 1-27.

Terrace, H. S. (1963b). Errorless transfer of a discrimination across two continua. *Journal of the Experimental Analysis of Behavior, 6,* 232 – 232.

Touchette, P. E. & Howard, J. S. (1984). Errorless learning: Reinforcement contingencies and stimulus control transfer in delayed prompting. *Journal of Applied Behavior Analysis, 17,* 175-188.

Chapter 4

COMPONENTS OF LANGUAGE TRAINING

Because language is such an essential and multi-faceted part of the curriculum it deserves a more detailed presentation. The following chapter will summarize some important concepts in teaching functional language to students. Although some authors are more comprehensive than others, most curricula containing language components address a number of similar core areas (e.g., Freeman & Dake, 1996; Larsson et al, 2000; Leaf & McEachin, 1999; Maurice, Green & Luce, 1996; Romanczyk, Lockshin, & Matey, 1996; Sundberg & Partington, 1998; Watson et al., 1989). The following general areas of instruction are usually included in a comprehensive language program and illustrate the extent of the task of teaching language:

- verbal imitation
- spontaneous language (mand and tact training)
- individual components of receptive and expressive communication
- mixing/generalizing individual components
- multiple-term sentences
- reciprocation
- conversation

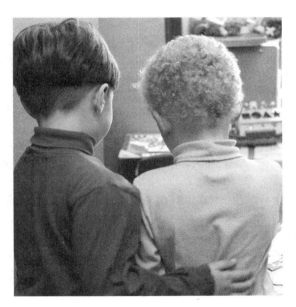

Many individual skills are subsumed under these basic headings but, hopefully, it is still clear from the list that the progression of skill acquisition from imitation through conversation is long and complex. Language is not simply the accumulation of a number of isolated skills. From the beginning there must be a focus on *spontaneous language* that occurs in a *natural environment*. It is the distinct goal of good language instruction to give the student language that is *functional* in the real world; this must be the foremost thought in the design and application of curricula.

Basic Language Concepts

The most fundamental and dominant concept in language is that words have the power to make things happen. This is crucial for the speaker because making things happen is the point of speaking. Children are born into the world without this power until they learn it, usually through a combination of engaging in behavior that comes naturally (making random sounds, imitating sounds and words in the environment, etc.) and the reinforcement that occurs for their sound-producing behavior (praise, attention, obtaining an object, etc.). Gradually, this sound-producing behavior gets shaped into words and sentences by parents, teachers, and peers.

If making sounds or saying words had no effect on the child or the child's environment *there would be few sounds or speech*. But since language has potent effects on the outside world, talking can come to be used by children (*function*) to obtain the things that they want. The first function or purpose to talking that appears in children is usually asking for things, first called *manding* by B. F. Skinner in his behavioral analysis of the development and function of language (Skinner, 1957).

Mands

A *mand* (think *de*-mand or *com*-mand) is language that requests something. Imagine a young child pointing to a cup of juice and saying, "That!" or "Ju." The function of the gesture/speech is to obtain the desired juice. The child might be able to simply pick up the cup of juice—in that case, there is no need for a mand and the child will probably engage in the simplest, most direct behavior—reaching for and picking up the cup. But, if the cup is out of reach, a mand to a parent for the juice may be necessary. The word *language* is used here in the broadest sense. A mand could be a sound, word, point, gesture, or any behavior used to communicate a desire for the juice.

Notice that mands are *social*—that is, they are directed at another person. Otherwise, they would not operate effectively. Think again of a child who says, "Ju" and points to a cup of juice on a table that is out of reach. If no one is in the room there is little chance that the child will obtain the juice and be reinforced for saying juice. Through the selective response of the environment, children learn to mand in the presence of others.

Tacts

A *tact* is language that labels an object present and in sight. A child looking up in the sky and, who, noticing an airplane, says, "plane" is tacting. The child is certainly not asking for someone to give him the airplane. The function of the behavior, then, must be different from requesting. Tacts are *mands for attention*. In the situation described above, the word "plane" is said so that a companion will respond socially ("Yes, that is an airplane!").

Intraverbals

An *intraverbal* is language that responds to the language of others, as when a student answers the question, "What's your name?" The main feature of the intraverbal is that the stimulus for a student's language is *other language* rather than a desire for objects or the attention of others. Much of everyday conversation is formed by intraverbals.

Receptive and Expressive Language

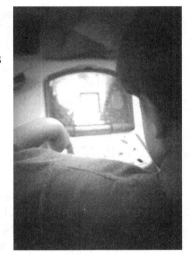

Receptive and *expressive* are terms used to describe two types of performances related to language. Most language has these two aspects. A receptive performance is one where a person listens to someone speak and then acts in some way related to what he or she just heard. For example, *following instructions* is usually a receptive task. The teacher says, "John, pick up the pencil" and John picks up the pencil. John does not speak but his behavior is based on what he has just heard.

Expressive performances are just the opposite. If the student gives the instruction, "Mrs. Brown, pick up the pencil" the student has engaged in an expressive performance. Likewise, with labeling, a teacher can say, "John, give me the block" and the student gives her the block (receptive) *or* the teacher can say, "What is this?" and the student can say, "block" (expressive). The following table contains some other examples of receptive and expressive performances.

Receptive Performance	Expressive Performance
"Point to Red" – (student points to red)	"What color" (student says, "red")
"Put the block *under*" – (student puts block under table)	"Where is the block" (student says, "under")
"Show me the big red clown under the table" - (Student picks out correct object)	"What's this?" (student says, "the big red clown is under the table")

Recap of Instructional Methodology

Language instruction follows the same general principles as other curriculum areas. Let's recap the main points:

1. Provide frequent opportunities for learning. Teach skills throughout the day in as many situations as possible. Arrange the environment to provide naturally occurring opportunities.

2. Arrange the task so that easier parts are learned first, in small easily performed bits. As much as possible make learning errorless

3. Use prompts to obtain a student performance if necessary but fade those prompts quickly

4. Generalize early. As soon as a new performance is consistently obtained in one setting, teach it in different settings and with different people

5. Mix individual drills as soon as they are mastered.

6. Pay attention to the child's self-initiated behavior. If the child wants or seems interested in something it can be an opportunity to teach.

7. Work towards a fluent, rapid performance, not just a performance that is correct eventually.

(*Note* that information related to *incidental teaching* is highly relevant to language instruction and is included in the next chapter.)

VERBAL IMITATION

It is imperative to begin as early as possible with mand training, even if a child is not imitating clearly or rapidly. In this way the child learns that speech (and verbal imitation) can be a powerful behavior in which to engage. If the student is not imitating verbally, other modes can be used to establish mands, tacts, and all the other forms of language. Picture communication systems (Frost & Bondy, 1994) and sign language (Sundberg & Partington, 1998) are two such methods. Sometimes the use of these systems creates an interest in communicating in the child that leads to verbal imitation and use of words. Other times the child continues to use the nonverbal communication system as the primary means of communicating.

A Word about Modeling Verbalizations

It is important to discuss what is actually modeled to the student to use as mands, tacts, and other verbalizations. Modeling occurs *often* and, therefore, it is crucial to do it correctly. *When we model we must say* exactly *what we want the student to say in a given situation.* With beginning students we do *not* add other directives or comments because that may distract or confuse the student. We do not say, "Say tickle;" we just say, "Tickle." This helps the student to avoid repeating the instruction part of the model. In addition, the model may be more easily faded in the future because there are fewer words to fade.

Table. Examples of Correct and Incorrect Verbal Models

Antecedents:	Do Not Say:	Say Instead:
A boy approaches, smiles, and holds up his arms. In the past he does this when he wants to be tickled.	"Say, I want a tickle"	"I want a tickle"
A girl picks up an empty cup and hands it to you.	"You want a drink? Say, drink"	"Drink"
A boy is looking out of a window at an approaching bus and jumping up and down with anticipation.	"It's time to go home, here's the bus. Can you say, 'Bus'?"	"I want to go home"

SPONTANEOUS LANGUAGE

Mands

Manding occurs in many ways, not just through words. Often, tantrums can be mands ("I want to go outside but you won't let me…" "I don't want to work") Aggression and self-injurious behavior can contain a message that is as clear as if the child had spoken. However, sometimes the nonverbal message is not at all clear or it would be inappropriate for caregivers to reinforce such problematic behavior. Usually, language is the best and most efficient way to make our needs and desires known to others. The specific words that a child requires are unique to each individual because their needs and desires are unique. However, many young children have a number of words in common: juice, on, up, tickle, play, go, down, etc. Simple observation is extremely helpful in determining what words are appropriate. When left to themselves in stimulating environments, children may manipulate, explore and interact with many things. Access to all of these interactions can be controlled by teaching personnel and awarded when appropriate language is given by the child.

Organize a Mand List

A comprehensive list arranged by setting is often helpful. This list can be easily made by following the child through the day and noting their interests and routines. Usually, the number of such opportunities to communicate wants or needs is vastly underestimated. Literally, hundreds of opportunities to mand exist every day; a beginning list should contain multiple mands for *each setting* in which the child spends time. Consider a few examples:

Environmental Event	Mand
New person in environment	"Play"
Sits on swing	"Push me"
Approaches TV	"On"
Approaches snack	"Goldfish"

Environmental Event (Continued)	Mand (Continued)
Picks up book	"Read to me"
Sees bus at end of day	"Time to go home"
Approaches refrigerator	"Juice"
Approaches parent/teacher	"Up"
Approaches door	"Out"
Looks at parent	"Tickle"
Looks at favorite toy out of reach	"Elmo"

A form to help organize a Mand List is included in the appendix.

Communication Temptations

Communication temptations are needs to use mands (or other language elements) that are created by teaching personnel, when these needs might not exist naturally (see also "contrived" learning opportunities in Chapter 5, Incidental Teaching). For example, when recess time arrives and the child wants to go outside, he or she could be required to say, "out" or "outside." After the word is produced the child might be told, "O.K., go get your coat." The child then runs to the closet to find an empty hanger. In such a situation the child can then learn to say, "Need coat" to teaching personnel. Communication temptations greatly increase the opportunities to use mands and other language.

Teaching Mands

Given a child who at least makes attempts to verbally imitate, the procedure to teach manding is straightforward. For children who do not verbally imitate, signs or pictures may be substituted for the words. The steps below apply to verbal mands or signs. See Frost & Bondy (1994) for details on a picture exchange system of manding. Remember that language training takes an enormous amount of work. No student would have enough time if learning depended only on time in scheduled classes or drills. Furthermore, manding serves a function—getting the person something. This happens according to the student's schedule, not the teacher's. Isolating practice to certain specific times tends to take the motivation out of practicing for the student. Mand training needs to occur all day, every day in order to establish it in the life of the student.

1. Wait for the child to show interest or need for something. This can either be naturally occurring or arranged by teaching personnel (communication temptations).

2. Withhold the desired object and model the mand.

3. Wait for the child to echo the verbalization (or imitate the sign).

4. If the child does not repeat the model within 2-3 seconds, continue modeling as needed waiting for 2-5 seconds in-between repetitions while redirecting the child's gaze to the object or activity to "tempt" them into talking. For signs, wait 2-3 seconds after the model sign and, if the model is not imitated, give physical prompts to perform the sign.

5. Immediately award the child with the desired object/event when an approximation of the mand is given.

6. Fade your model in the future after a few strong responses from the student. For verbal mands, first try directing the student to the object/activity and then waiting for 2 seconds. If no response from the student try the first letter of the word. If no response, give the entire word. *Make sure that the child says the entire word before getting the object/event* rather than repeating just the partial prompt of the model. For signs fade the physical prompts to brief touches or partial models of the correct sign before eliminating the prompts altogether.

Get the Momentum Going

Reinforcing events can be manipulated to help evoke language. Imagine holding out a hand to a student in a playful way, saying, "High five" and tickling the student after he slaps your hand. Repeat the action several times and the child may become excited and more strongly seek the tickle, trying hard to do the "High five." Before delivering the next tickle, you can model a mand ("tickle") and wait for the child to imitate. The child is now more likely to imitate the mand to obtain the tickle because the reinforcer has been well established, creating the momentum to continue. Fun activities like this could also include swinging the child around ("swing me"), pushing the child on a swing ("push"), or chasing the child ("chase me"). In each case the activity is begun by engaging in the activity several times. When the child is completely engaged an additional requirement is added.

Eye Contact

Sometimes, eye contact with the teacher or parent naturally accompanies requests. Other times eye contact develops after the child is regularly and spontaneously asking for items. If eye contact is not given with requests even after the child regularly asks for a few things, the adult can try delaying a response to the request. This "unexpected" response may prompt the child to repeat the request with more intensity, including looking at the adult. If delayed responding does not produce eye contact, a more individualized strategy may be necessary to prompt eye contact. *Shared attention activities* may be extremely helpful in establishing spontaneous eye contact. See Chapter 6 – *Social Interaction and Integration.*

Teaching Tacts

Sometimes, after a number of mands have been taught the child is often ready to learn tacting (also called commenting). Note that the same methodologies used to teach manding can be employed to establish tacts, with the student learning to spontaneously name things, events, and people around him or her. The most frequent reinforcer for tacting is social approval from the person who accompanies the student. If a student says "car" when looking at a bright red car, the logical response from the "environment" should be for those around the child to acknowledge the verbalization ("Yes, that's a car! Wow, you like cars? I do too."). If this reaction is reinforcing to the child, tacting "car" will probably increase. Alternatively, if praise and an enthusiastic reaction is not enough, other forms of reinforcement can be delivered to increase tacting, like bits of edibles, tickles, or tokens.

Walks in interesting environments, looking at fun books, listening to stimulating songs, and watching favorite videos are all ways to make certain things in the environment more prominent. When the student's attention is drawn to the object, person, or feature of the environment, they can be given a model prompt to name it. If they learn that some form of reinforcement will be delivered for their naming they often begin to spontaneously name the things in their environment. Time must be allocated for these activities in the student's schedule, with a list of words to be taught created for different settings. Start slowly with just a few words and start in highly motivating settings. Fade the model prompts in the same way that models were faded for mands.

Let's illustrate teaching tacts with a hypothetical situation. Dan is a four-year-old boy who has about 25 spontaneous mands. He freely gives eye contact and enjoys social interactions with adults. He especially likes to take walks around the hallways of the school. In his cubby, his instructional assistant has worked with him on identifying common objects (pointing to them in response to the IA's request, "Show me apple") and also in naming the objects ("What's this?" "Apple"). He has mastered about 30 labels in this setting. Lately, Dan has responded more to the talking of others around him, repeating bits of what they are saying.

Dan's ABA consultant, teacher, and instructional assistant have decided to begin a program to increase labeling of things in the natural environment during walks around the school. They have identified 10 different objects that Dan looks at during these walks and have these words listed in his program book. During 15-minute sessions, two times per day, the IA and Dan walk in the hallways practicing tacts. First, the IA stops Dan in front of a big picture of a clown that Dan loves. As soon as he approaches and looks at it, she says "Clown." Dan hesitates while looking at the picture. Three seconds later the IA repeats, "Clown" and Dan says "Cown." The IA exclaims, "Yes! What a great clown. [tickles Dan] Good job, Clown." Next, they walk around the halls naming the list of other objects that Dan likes. After two or three times, Dan is starting to anticipate the objects on his route through the halls. As he comes around one particular corner he now runs to the picture on the wall and *yells* "Clown" (the IA now has to work on not yelling!).

Because Dan is getting the hang of labeling and understanding that he will be rewarded by the IA for tacting, he is starting to name things in other environments. The IA has started adding labels of things in other environments, according to what seems to interest Dan. In addition, a list of objects at home has been established.

ESTABLISHING INDIVIDUAL COMPONENTS

Before a student is able to run they must walk. Before a student talks in sentences they learn to use single words. An excellent list of individual drills for teaching receptive and expressive language is contained in the curriculum of The Autism Partnership (Leaf & McEachin, 1999). There are numerous target skills ranging from labeling simple discriminations (colors, shapes, attributes, etc.) to complex relationships between objects or people, or multi-step performances (discussing past events, telling a story, etc.). A few examples of individual components include:

- Receptive/Expressive Labels
- Receptive Instructions
- Attributes (color, size, features, construction)
- Yes/no
- Functions of objects
- Categories
- Answering Wh-questions (who, what, when, where, why)
- Same/different
- Prepositions
- Pronouns
- Emotions
- Before/after
- First/last
- Past and future verb tenses
- Plurals
- Recalling past events
- Telling stories
- Cause and effect

It is not desirable to wait for all of these performances to be developed before proceeding to other aspects of training like generalization or multiple term sentences (see below). However, individual components must be mastered *individually* before they may be combined with other components in longer, more complex sentences. Thus, a child must be able to name a ball ("ball") before he or she is asked to describe the ball ("blue ball," "big, blue ball"). As soon as a few individual components are taught they can be combined, both receptively and expressively and, as newer additional components are taught they can be added to the mix to form longer sentences.

Sentence Stems

If a student is spontaneously manding and tacting it may be time to ask for phrases and sentences. One place to start is to ask the student to use *sentence stems*. These are groups of words that can begin many sentences:

- "I want a …"
- "I see a …"
- "That's a …"
- "I have a …"

+ "There's a …"
+ "It's a …"
+ "I am …"

The child learns the formula for different kinds of sentences by using a particular stem with various endings. Of course, the student should start with one stem (usually, "I want …") and add others only as previous stems are mastered. Once the child shows that they can spontaneously use the stems in combination with various objects and events, teaching personnel should require the entire sentence before responding. Consistency in this regard is very important.

Teachers should be aware that a child who uses sentence stems does not necessarily understand the grammar involved or even the meaning of the individual words like "I" or "see." In the beginning "I want a cookie" is just a longer version of "cookie." Later, when the child learns pronouns, the significance of "I", "you", "he", and "she" will be understood but only then. Until then, view the use of sentence stems as no more than fancier versions of simple tacts and mands that are designed to sound better (more grammatically correct) to listeners.

MIXING AND GENERALIZING INDIVIDUAL COMPONENTS

As individual components of speech are learned they are integrated into daily speech. This is first established with the mand list. Then, the student is asked to start naming (tacting) the things or people in their environments. While the student is becoming better at this, individual component performances like those listed in the previous section are established. Usually, this teaching would be done as isolated drills, depending on the target skill and materials needed. As soon as the child begins to learn the skills, however, they are slowly added to the growing group of skills implemented in the natural environment and presented in a mixed fashion. As with mixing drills in a discrete trial format, the child works on one or two trials of one drill, one trial of another drill, two trials of a third, one trial again of the first drill, etc. By mixing the drills together the student must pay close attention to what is asked. Furthermore, performing the drills in a natural setting helps the student learn to use the skills throughout the day.

Sundberg and Partington (1999) describe a way to organize the mix of some of the receptive drills, called *receptive by feature, function, and class (RFFC)*. In this procedure the student is asked alternately to identify objects by their attributes (feature), their purpose (function), or their category (class). For example:

"Touch the one that you eat with." (function)
"Touch the one that is red" (feature)
"Touch the one that is long" (feature)
"Touch the one that is jumping" (feature)
"Touch the one that is an animal" (class)

Notice that the student is not asked to name anything. All of these drills are done receptively. Later, other drills can be added that include expressive language drills as well.

MULTIPLE TERM SENTENCES

When the child has a basic repertoire of tacts and mands he or she can begin to combine these elements into what are called *multiple term* sentences. A term is one element of a sentence. Larsson (2000) lists seven basic elements:

- Subject
- Object
- Action
- Preposition
- Adjective
- Pronoun
- Possessive pronoun

When the elements are combined in the various possible ways the following performances are produced, called a *two-term sentence*:

Combination of elements:	Example
Subject/Action	"Tiger run"
Subject/Preposition	"Elephant on top"
Object/Preposition	"Wagon behind"
Action/Object	"Throw ball"
Pronoun/Action	"She walk"
Preposition/Object	"In box"
Adjective/Subject	"Big boy"
Adjective/Object	"Tall building"
Pronoun/Action	"He run"
Possessive Pronoun/Object	"Her shirt"

The elements can also be combined to make three, four, and five term sentences. Each combination is taught receptively *and* expressively. Larsson suggests that each combination should be taught using 2D stimuli (pictures), 3D stimuli, on the child's body, on the staff's body, using written materials, and when used in everyday situations or stories.

RECIPROCATION AND CONVERSATION

Even though a student is able to spontaneously describe the environment in fairly complex ways their speech will not resemble normal conversation unless there is a *reciprocal* quality to it. This means that each participant in the conversation takes turns in making statements and asking questions related to what the other person says.

Speaker 1	Speaker 2
"How are you?"	"I'm fine. How are you?"
"I'm fine. What did you do at lunch?"	"I played with Teddy. What did you do?"
"I had pizza with Jason. It was yucky!"	"Yeah, I hate this pizza! (giggles) Want to play on the swings?"
"O.K."	"Let's go!"

In contrast to answering questions with statements, the student must learn that there are times when they should respond to a statement with another statement. This type of training may be completely new to the student.

Speaker 1	Speaker 2
"I have a green shirt"	"I have a blue shirt"
"I like bananas"	"I like apples"
"My name is Shawn"	"My name is Lisa"

Once a person learns to reciprocate a statement with another statement, more complicated interactions can be taught. Reciprocation has several basic performances that can be taught individually including:

Speaker 1	Speaker 2
Statement/Question	
"I have a green shirt."	"Where did you get it?"
Statement/Negative Statement	
"I like bananas."	"I don't like bananas."
Statement/Statement/Question	
: "I like apples."	"I like hotdogs. Do you like hotdogs too?"

Note that in the beginning conversations taught above, questions form one important element. Sometimes before questions can be integrated into conversations they may need to be explicitly taught. The following are examples of questions that should be included in the curriculum. (Note that the student should learn to ask the questions of *others* rather than respond to the questions.)

- **What is it/What's that?**
- **Who is it?**
- **Where is it**
- **What are you doing?**
- **What's in there?**
- **Where are you going?**

✦ **Who has it?**

✦ **What's wrong?**

The skill of asking questions must generalize to natural environments so that questions are used spontaneously. As with other language elements, in order to accomplish this, the environment should be arranged so that asking questions becomes *necessary*, *frequent*, and *functional*. For example, at dismissal, the child finds his coat missing and must say, "Where is my coat?" At lunch the child's food tray is not delivered and she must say, "Where's my lunch?" The child is told, "Someone has a treat for you" and must ask, "Who has it?" Like all other aspects of language learned, asking questions is immediately reinforced and gradually extended to all of the child's environments as well as added to conversations.

By the time language training reaches an advanced level, children may be picking up language from many sources (peers, T.V., adult conversations), throughout the day, both in 1:1 interactions and in groups. At this stage access to peers, social opportunities, and active groups of many kinds is crucial. Advanced language concepts in curriculums include getting and giving information in groups, role-taking, and making inferences. Certain settings may require specific subject-related language. However, the fundamentals of language acquisition will still need to be recalled. Language must be *functional* and *required* by the environment if it is to survive and increase. Students must be given frequent opportunities to use language and be reinforced.

Key Concepts and Questions

1. Define the terms *mand, tact, intraverbal*.

2. Give an example of receptive and expressive language.

3. When modeling or prompting verbalizations what should be modeled and what should not be modeled?

4. What is a *mand list* and why create one?

5. What are *communication temptations* and provide examples?

6. Describe how to teach mands.

7. How often should language training occur?

8. Name some *individual components* of the language curriculum that might be taught in isolation first.

9. Give two examples of *sentence stems*.

10. Why are language drills mixed after they are mastered separately?

11. What is RFFC?

12. Name the seven basic elements of a sentence, according to Larsson.

13. Give an example of a two-term sentence using Action/Object.

14. Give an example of a three-term sentence using Subject/Action/Object.

15. Give an example of reciprocation performance where a student responds to a statement with another statement.

16. Explain the following statement: "In order to teach students to ask questions, the environment should be arranged so that asking questions becomes necessary, frequent, and functional."

References and Resources

Freeman, S. & Dake, B. A. (1997). Teach Me Language. Langley, British Columbia, CA: SKF Books, 20641 46th Avenue, Langley, B.C., Canada V3A 3H8.

Frost, L.A., & Bondy, A. S. (1994). *The Picture Exchange Communication System Training Manual.* Cherry Hill, NJ: Pyramid Educational Consultants, Inc.

Larsson, E., (2000) The Language Matrix. Workshop given at the annual convention of the Association for Behavior Analysis, May 26, 2000.

Leaf, R. & McEachin, J. (Eds.) (1999). *A Work in Progress.* New York, NY: DRL Books (800) 853-1057; www.drlbooks.com

Maurice, C., Green, G., & Luce, S. (1996). *Behavioral Intervention for Young Children with Autism.* Austin, TX: Pro-Ed, (800) 897-3202; www.proedinc.com

Romanczyk, R. G., Lockshin, S. & Matey, L. (1996). *Individualized Goal Selection Curriculum.* Apalachin, NY: Clinical Behavior Therapy Associates, Suite 5, 3 Tioga Boulevard, Apalachin, NY 13732, (607) 625-4438.

Skinner, B. F. (1957). Verbal Behavior. Acton, MA: Copley Publishing Group, Acton, MA 01720.

Sundberg, M. L. & Partington, J. W. (1998). Teaching Language to Children with Autism or Other Developmental Disabilities. Pleasant Hill, CA: Behavior Analysts, Inc. 3329 Vincent Road, Pleasant Hill, CA 94526.

Watson, L. R., Lord, C., Schaffer, B. & Schopler, E. (1989). *Teaching Spontaneous Communication to Autistic and Developmentally Handicapped Children.* Austin, TX: Pro-Ed, (800) 897-3202; www.proedinc.com

Chapter 5

INCIDENTAL TEACHING

>*On the way to Grandmother's house two children sit in the back seat of a Buick playing* I Spy. *"I spy something red," says the 8-year-old girl and her 6-year-old brother launches into a series of guesses as to the identity of the red something.*

From the perspective of the children, the language game is *incidental* to the main reason for being in the car—of course; they are going to Grandmother's house. Their game-related actions (secretly choosing objects, giving clues, making guesses) are, in some ways, external to the chain of behaviors leading to Grandmother (getting ready, walking to the car, riding in the car, getting out of the car). The game is a brief interlude that is inserted into the main activity, with its own set of actions and motivations.

In this section we will discuss the nature and techniques of teaching incidentally. We will distinguish it from other forms of teaching, discuss the underlying learning processes involved, illustrate the techniques in some real-world cases, identify target behaviors that are appropriate for incidental teaching, and make recommendations for implementation and usage.

Why Teach Incidentally?

Incidental teaching has been recommended by practitioners for inclusion in ABA programs for several reasons. Lovaas (1982) advocated incidental teaching in order to help *make every minute of the student's day educational.* He recommended the presentation of discrete trial sessions interspersed with play breaks, with the advice that play should be made as educational as possible. Teaching incidentally in a natural environment has been suggested as promoting generalization and spontaneous use of learned skills (Hart & Risley, 1980).

Other authors have discussed the advantages of incidental teaching as *motivational* (Michael, 1988; Sundberg, 1993), pointing out that, in non-directive environments, the stimuli with which students choose to engage can be, potentially, more powerful reinforcers than those that might be chosen in advance by a teacher. Teachers can identify and co-opt these preferred stimuli, or what Sundberg calls to "...*capture* or *contrive* the reinforcing effectiveness of an event" in order to effect a behavior change (1993, P. 211). For example, an incidental learning opportunity may begin with a teacher noticing that a child approaches a toy. Before gaining possession of it, the child could be required by the teacher to imitate the name of the toy (capturing motivation). Or, an adult may stand in front of a video blocking the view until a child says, "Move, please" (contriving motivation). Interrupting the acquisition of a desirable toy or the viewing of a video allows the teacher to require the student to incidentally perform a new skill and creates a situation where continuation of the previous activity reinforcers the performance of the new skill. This methodology is known as incidental teaching. Note, especially, that since the student's self-initiated behavior (in the form of approach, interest, and engagement with stimuli) is often the most reliable signal that a particular stimulus may be eligible to act as a reinforcer, successful incidental teaching opportunities may depend on close observation and identification of such motivation-related events. Once identified the events may be arranged or manipulated so that access by the student only follows the emission of specified target behavior(s).

The strategy of identifying reinforcers through observing *child-initiated actions* and using them to prompt and consequate target behaviors is a powerful use of incidental teaching. A student who is poorly motivated and inattentive in more structured settings may require delivery of much of their program in an environment where *they choose most of the activities in which they engage* and, therefore, spend much of their time in the "natural environment." In a teacher-directed environment (such as discrete trials) self-initiated behavior and choice may not always be appropriate. As seen earlier, in discrete trials, a student would be expected to respond to teacher-directed activities followed by teacher-chosen consequences. This may be difficult for some students, especially those who are very young or inexperienced with more structured learning settings.

Use of the term "natural environment" is not meant here to imply that some environments are *not* natural. Settings differ in various respects, making them different in their suitability for teaching purposes. The use of incidental teaching in a child-directed environment should be differentiated from other locations of incidental teaching. Incidental teaching may be used *both* in settings where child-initiated actions are frequent or where they are not prominent. In fact, although incidental teaching is often discussed as occurring in certain environments (Fenske, Krantz, & McClannahan, 2001), its location may not be central to its definition at all. Incidental teaching mainly implies that there is an activity most prominent or central at the moment for the student, the continuation of which serves as a reinforcer for engaging in another (incidental) activity. This may occur in child or adult-directed environments. For example, while teaching a child to brush her teeth a parent might hold up the toothbrush and ask, "What's this?" before going on. The parent is attempting to use the continuation of the activity of tooth brushing to reinforce the student for answering the inserted question. Any activity in which there is a high probability of engagement and continued participation may serve to reinforce engagement in lower probability (incidental) behavior, regardless of who initiates the high probability activity. This is referred to as the *Premack Principle* (Premack, 1959).

Illustrations of incidental teaching are provided below. Note that some published curricula incorporate specific strategies that depend on inducing motivation, including advice and examples of arranging an environment and specific teacher actions to stimulate the use of spontaneous language (such as the area "Communication Temptations" in Leaf & McEachin (1999), the section on "Engineering the Environment" in Watson et al. (1989), or the "natural environment training" of Sundberg & Partington (1998)).

Examples of Incidental Teaching

Jenn was a six-year-old girl with a diagnosis of PDD-NOS who received an ABA program for 32 hours per week comprised of a variety of educational activities. Several times per day she was encouraged to play in an area of the room where there were many shelves with interesting activities and games. Jenn tended to choose puzzles every time she played and Jenn's teaching assistant wanted to help her to branch out into more elaborate kinds of play. One day before play time the TA put Jenn's favorite puzzles in a cupboard hidden from sight. When Jenn went to the shelf where the puzzles were normally kept and did not see them, she spent a few seconds looking around the area for them. At this point the TA approached Jenn and said, "Where are the puzzles?" Jenn replied, "I don't know" and continued to look in the general area. Picking up and placing a puppet of Elmo on her hand the TA began to move the puppet around, pretending to look for the puzzles and narrating as she went along. "Well, let's see, they aren't in *here*. Nope, not here either…" Jenn looked over at the puppet as the TA continued. As soon as Jenn looked in her direction, the TA took off the puppet and put it on Jenn's hand, saying, "You make it look!" Using a few brief touch prompts the TA prompted Jenn to begin the search. Jenn moved the puppet around but did not talk. "I don't hear Elmo saying anything," called the TA, and Jenn began saying "Not here" with some movements. Although Jenn complied, it was clear that she was merely complying with the TA's instructions because her actions were brief and cursory, and she looked at the TA for approval often. As Jenn's attention flagged, in order to hasten discovery of the puzzles (and, thus, reinforcement), the TA pointed to the cupboard with the puzzles and said; "Look in here." Jenn moved to the cupboard, making the puppet open the door with the puppet's mouth, and saw her favorite puzzles. She immediately took off the puppet, seized the puzzles and began to play with them.

In subsequent play sessions the TA continued to hide the puzzles and Jenn reenacted the search with the puppet. Each time, the TA required a bit more pretend play and more elaborate language. The puppet eventually walked, flew, was tired, made funny noises, commented on various things, and narrated what other people were doing— all during the search for the puzzles.

Peter did not use language to communicate with others but he did repeat what others said in rough approximations. During lunch he ate an assortment of foods and drank milk (his favorite) from a cup. Peter's teacher wanted to increase Peter's communication skills, so she decided to begin with teaching him to ask for the items he wanted at lunch. One day she sat next to him while he ate and held onto the cup of milk. When he reached for it she moved it slightly away and said, "Milk." Peter repeated, "Milk" and the teacher immediately said, "Good! Milk" gave him the cup, and allowed him a sip. Taking possession of the cup again, the teacher waited until Peter reached for it again. "Mi— " said the teacher" and Peter said, "Mi—." "Milk" corrected the teacher and Peter said, "Milk," again receiving the cup. On the third try Peter repeated "Milk" after just a prompt of the initial sound. On the fourth try Peter said "Milk" when the cup was held up by the teacher. The names of all of the foods that Peter routinely ate were taught in the same way.

Some time later, the teacher removed the cup from the table before sitting next to Peter during lunch. After a few bites Peter began looking for his cup but did not find it. The teacher brought out an empty cup, holding it so that Peter could plainly see that no milk was in it. "Cup" she said, and Peter said, "Cup." "Great, here's a cup" said the teacher, giving him the cup, and immediately bringing out an 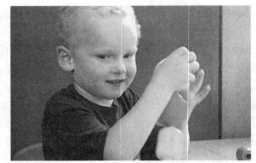 open carton of milk, showing it to him and waiting. After a silence of two seconds, she prompted, "M—" and Peter said, "Milk." The teacher praised Peter and immediately poured the milk. After he drank the small amount of milk, the teacher took back the cup and put it out of sight again. Within a short time Peter was asking for the cup if it wasn't present, followed by a request for milk. Eventually he set his place at the lunch table by asking for a list of things, including "plate," "cup," 2 utensils, and a number of foods; in addition, he used several action verbs as instructions to the teacher (open, more, give me, help), and chose a preferred food using a name ("What do you want, spaghetti or mustard?"). This success encouraged the teacher to begin to integrate receptive language tasks into the mealtime that had been mastered in discrete trials ("Point to red" on a box with a picture of the colors of a rainbow). Sometimes the teacher put Peter's small toy figures on the table and asked him to make the figures do things like jump, sleep, fly, etc. During the meal the teacher was careful that Peter spent enough time eating; interruptions for incidental activities were brief and spaced apart so that Peter did not become frustrated.

Twice a day **Willy** engaged in an activity with his Instructional Assistant that the consultant calls the "Drill Dump." The target performances for this activity came from all of the individual skill programs that Willy had mastered at his cubby (a considerable list of 5 pages). Whenever a drill was mastered in discrete trials it was added to the list. Willy could already follow mixed instructions from this list at the table in his cubby (see the sections on mixed drills in the previous chapters). The IA would bring Willy out into the common area of the classroom, into another activity area, or even out on the playground and begin a fun activity. During the activity the IA briefly interrupted Willy to ask questions but monitored Willy carefully in order to choose the right time to require a particular behavior. For example, the IA noticed that if he waits for Willy to approach an object, it is easier to get a response to a question involving the object.

Sandra loved engaging in arts and crafts activities. Her teacher decided to set up an arts & crafts activity every day so that she could work on various skills like following instructions, more advanced expressive language, spontaneous commenting, and asking for help. The teacher integrated the skills into the activity, so that Sandra had to engage in the target behaviors in order to continue to complete the activity.

Susan was learning to comment on things in her environment but was somewhat shy about talking spontaneously. Since Susan loved to walk around the school her paraprofessional decided to try and teach comments incidentally during daily excursions. During these walks the paraprofessional waited for Susan to show an interest in something and then ran up to it, exclaiming "I see a (name of object)!" She then looked at Susan and waited for Susan to echo her comment. Sometimes she had to tap the object and repeat her comment a few times, looking back at Susan but, eventually, Susan echoed the comment, which was followed by enthusiastic agreement, smiling, and pats on the back from the paraprofessional. The paraprofessional and Susan then continued on with their walk to the next station. Following the same route around the school every day resulted in Susan adopting these comments and spontaneously uttering them when she came into the area. She seemed to enjoy the reaction she got from the paraprofessional. In a few cases when Susan ran up to something new, the paraprofessional simply pointed to the object and Susan spontaneously said, "I see a (name of object)!"

Discussion of Examples

In all of the preceding examples the students were engaged in a primary activity that was motivating, with built-in elements that could be manipulated in order to provide reinforcement for engaging in secondary or incidental tasks presented by an adult. Some activities occurred naturally, others were arranged by teaching personnel but all engaged the student fully. Access to and continuation of the activity was highly desirable to the student and, therefore, provided the motivation for completing a few "extra," incidental tasks. The examples illustrate how simple incidental tasks can be built upon to make more complex and lengthy chains of performances without disturbing the primary activity. Certainly, if the primary activity is interrupted for a long period of time with many difficult extra steps, the distance of the incidental tasks from the reinforcer (the primary activity) increases and the likelihood that the incidental performance will be supported and maintained decreases. However, if initial incidental requirements are brief and new behavior is slowly added, the weight of the added incidental tasks may be more easily sustained.

Organizing Incidental Teaching

While it may be a highly effective teaching format, incidental teaching is also among the most difficult to implement logistically. Unfortunately, this is probably inherent in the nature of the format. Incidental teaching is not the primary activity in a particular setting and, therefore, may receive less emphasis from instructors or those organizing the curriculum. It may also seem at first glance that incidental teaching is difficult to schedule—that it occurs between or around scheduled activities and, therefore, its occurrence is variable and dependent. However, some rethinking and analysis of the task (i.e., what behavior analysts do best!) may help.

Incidental teaching always occurs at *some* time, that is, during some activity like car rides, recess on the playground, lunchtime, walks, etc. In each setting or activity a specific repertoire of skills is relevant and tied to the unique learning goals of the student.

By analyzing the setting-specific required skills, student abilities, and present goals, a set of *primary* and *incidental* target behaviors can be specified for each activity or setting. For example, during a car ride, the primary activity requires a child to walk to the car, open the door, climb up on the seat, close the door, buckle the seat-belt, and wait for arrival at the destination. Incidental skills required during the car ride would be specific to the abilities of the child but might include asking for a book or other activity, commenting on the sights that pass, or answering questions about surroundings and the destination.

Organizing incidental teaching into settings, primary, and incidental skills can help teachers focus on specific objectives. An example of this kind of organization is provided in the following table.

Table: Example of organizing primary and incidental skills by setting.

This form is included in the appendix.

Setting/Activity	Category	Current Target Behaviors:
Playground	Primary Skills	**Slide**: climbs up slide and slides down independently **Swings**: sits on swing while being pushed for 2 minutes **Run**: runs on uneven surfaces **Chase Game**: approaches peer and says, "chase me." Runs away when peer chases. **Soccer**: kicks ball and runs after it in a group of peers
	Incidental Skills	**Receptive/expressive Labels**: locates and goes to various toys and items of playground equipment or answers question from adult, "What is this?" **Receptive/Expressive Labels**: locates and goes to person named or answers question from adult, "Who is this?" **Imitation in a series**: follows prompts to imitate a series of actions related to a game. **Making a choice**: Answers question, "What do you want to do?" by naming activity and using the sentence stem: "I want to…" **Making comments**: Gets attention of typical peer or adult by pointing to something and saying, "I see a _____." **Prepositions**: follows one sentence instructions involving play equipment and prepositions or positioning self in relation to objects (e.g., "Put the shovel *in* the pail" or "Go *under* the slide").
Lunch/Snack	Primary Skills	**Pouring**: pours milk from carton into cup independently without causing cup to overflow. **Eating**: unwraps sandwich and eats independently **Cutting with fork**: uses fork to cut/separate larger pieces of food when hot lunch is served **Clean up**: throws out garbage, puts dirty dishes in sink, wipes placemat, and puts placemat away, independently.
	Incidental Skills	**Spontaneous Requests**: asks for needed items when not present (lunch, utensils, cup) and asks for more milk. **Making comments**: gets attention of typical peer or adult by pointing to something and saying, "I see a _____." **Receptive/Expressive Color**: points to or names color of indicated object at table **Prepositions:** follows instruction involving objects at table and prepositions. **Receptive/Expressive Labels/Functions**: locates cup and utensils or answers question from adult, "What is this?" and "What do you do with it?"

Organizing Incidental Language Instruction

MacDuff, Krantz, MacDuff, & McClannahan (1988) advocate data collection of student and instructor behavior as a way to promote and evaluate incidental teaching of language. They provide an example of a data sheet that records each child-initiated verbalization for an item or activity and whether an instructor responded with a prompt, model, or request for elaborated speech. Since data on staff as well as student behavior is collected, use of the form in incidental settings can be helpful as a staff training tool as well as an evaluation of a student's behavior. An adapted version of the form is pictured below. Six categories of student verbal behavior are listed (mands, tacts, verbal imitation, intraverbals, vocalizations, and jargon/echolalia). The observer records an entry for each student's verbal or vocal response, assigning a category and marking the code in the box marked "student." For each student behavior an antecedent (spontaneous, verbally prompted, communication temptation created by teacher) and all consequences (purposely ignored, prompt to refine pronunciation, prompt to lengthen utterance, reinforced by teacher) are recorded in corresponding boxes.

In addition to the codes, a more detailed record (i.e., the specific words or sentences used by the student) can be recorded on the data sheet if desired but much information is available from just calculating the rate of verbalizations, the proportion of verbalizations that are spontaneous vs. prompted, and the frequency of various consequences delivered by the instructor. Initial use of the form with new staff members usually requires detailed discussion of the results combined with suggestions from a more experienced teacher for improving the new instructor's effective use of prompts and reinforcers. This is an important benefit to use of the form because incidental settings are typically less structured than other settings and tend to be more difficult settings for instructors to recognize and maintain frequent teaching opportunities. In addition, ongoing use allows the student's language instruction in non-drill settings to be monitored and documented.

This form is included in the appendix.

Incidental Language Data Sheet

Student Behavior
M = Mands
T = Tacts
VI = Verbal Imitation
I = Intraverbal
VOC = Vocalization (not word)
J = Jargon/Echolalia

Antecedents (choose one)
S = Spontaneous
VP = Verbally Prompted
CT = Communication Temptation Created by Teacher

Consequences: (note all that are delivered)
IG = Purposely Ignored to Encourage Closer Approximation
R = Model Prompt Given to Refine Pronunciation
L = Longer Utterance Required
R+ = Reinforced by teacher

Instructions: categorize each utterance of the student using the labels above and write the code in the first blank box below marked "student" (working downwards). For each student utterance choose from the list above the antecedent and consequences observed and write the corresponding code in the box marked "teacher."

Date: _____   Instructor: _____

Location/Activity: _____

Start Time: _____   Observer: _____

Student	Antecedent	Consequences	Student	Antecedent	Consequences

As the student's language skills develop beyond saying the first few words and the organization of language instruction in natural settings becomes more complicated, it may be helpful to write down the words and phrases that the student recognizes or says.

Combined with current target words and phrases, *word lists* can provide implementers with easily accessible reference materials with which to keep their knowledge of the child's verbal abilities up to date. This is especially important when there are implementers that may not work with the child every day or work with her in different settings like the home or a therapy room.

Summary

While incidental teaching has been described as teaching in the "natural" environment this description alone may not adequately explain the important principles that make incidental teaching so valuable. The effectiveness of incidental teaching comes from the availability of a highly motivating primary activity, which is used to reinforce required new behavior, briefly inserted into the activity. Because the technique is fundamentally concerned with reinforcement, it is not surprising that it can be extremely useful for teaching students with autism. The logistics of arranging incidental teaching may be difficult and structuring it according to settings or activities may be helpful. Appropriate primary and incidental skills can be listed for each setting or activity that will help implementers focus on specific targets. Data collection on student and instructor behavior in incidental settings may also provide useful feedback to help increase the frequency and quality of learning opportunities and document student progress.

Key Concepts and Questions

1. Give two reasons for teaching incidentally.
2. While teaching in a natural environment may be one example of incidental teaching, this chapter states that incidental teaching may also occur during structured teaching. Give an example.
3. Give an example of a primary activity and skills incidental to that activity.
4. How would reinforcement be "captured or contrived?"
5. Describe the logic behind organizing incidental teaching according to setting or activity.

References and Resources

Fenske, E. C., Krantz, P. J., & McClannahan, L. E. (2001). Incidental Teaching: A Not-Discrete-Trial Teaching Procedure. In Maurice, C., Green, G., & Foxx, R. M. (2001). *Making a Difference, Behavioral Intervention for Autism.* Austin, TX: Pro-ed.

Hart, B., & Risley, T. R. (1980). *How to Use Incidental Teaching for Elaborating Language.* Lawrence, KS: H & H Enterprises, Inc.

Leaf, R. & McEachin, J. (Eds.) (1999). *A Work in Progress.* New York, NY: DRL Books (800) 853-1057; www.drlbooks.com

Lovaas, O. I. (1982). *Teaching Developmentally Disabled Children: The ME Book.* Austin, TX: Pro-Ed.

MacDuff, G. S., Krantz, P. J., MacDuff, M. A., & McClannahan, L. E. (1988). Providing incidental teaching for autistic children: a rapid training procedure for therapists. *Education and Treatment of Children, 11,* pp. 205-217.

Michael, J. (1988). Establishing operations and the mand. *The Analysis of Verbal Behavior, 6,* P. 3 – 9.

Premack, D. (1959). Toward empirical behavioral laws: I. Positive reinforcement. *Psychological Review, 66,* P. 219 – 233.

Sundberg, M. L. (1993). The application of establishing operations. *The Behavior Analyst, 16,* P. 211 – 214.

Sundberg, M. L. & Partington, J. W. (1998). *Teaching Language to Children with Autism or Other Developmental Disabilities.* Pleasant Hill, CA: Behavior Analysts, Inc. 3329 Vincent Road, Pleasant Hill, CA 94526.

Watson, L. R., Lord, C., Schaffer, B., & Schopler, E. (1989). *Teaching Spontaneous Communication to Autistic and Developmentally Handicapped Children.* Austin, TX: Pro-ed.

Chapter 6

SOCIAL INTERACTION AND INTEGRATION

In order for a student to become a member of a peer group in a classroom, on a playground, or at a family gathering, the skills necessary to interact with other group members must be acquired. Group members *initiate* and *respond* to each other as well as *participate* in determining the structure of the interaction. In other words, peers themselves decide when and how to interact rather than following prompts from an external leader. In addition to the structure, the source of reinforcement in peer-led interactions is usually different from adult-led activities. Rather than acting out of a desire for tangible rewards or praise from an adult, the reinforcement is usually at least partially social and intrinsic to the activity. For these reasons peer-initiated and structured interactions are different in some respects from other kinds of interactions. For example, on the playground children choose their play partners, initiating and responding to social "bids" (invitations to play) from others. Once chosen, during ongoing interactions, the group members determine the specific activities in which they will engage, including the length, location, pace, and contingencies of reinforcement and punishment. Two athletic boys may pair up and start running around a play apparatus, up the ladder, down the slide, through the tunnel, past the swings, and back again. Others observe and decide to join the fun, joining a line of runners. Some participants overtake the leader and take the group in a different direction. The group members bump into each other, laughing and shouting. Various members initiate gross motor actions like waving their arms or vocalizations like making zoom noises that are imitated by others. Finally, exhausted, the leaders fall on the grass and those behind follow suit. After a pause of a few moments, the group breaks into several pairs or trios that converse until they are ready for more action.

In young children, *peer-initiated and structured activities* probably occur most commonly in various types of social play activities. However, the basic components of social play are often learned in isolation from others. For example, some children may learn to throw or bounce a ball, run, climb, build towers, roll trucks, or ride a bike by themselves. This does not mean that they automatically begin to engage in these activities with others. Early in their social development students need to sample the various types of social interactions and may require a great deal of interaction with others before they spontaneously seek it. They may not naturally tend towards "shared" or "joint attention" experiences, preferring to isolate themselves and avoid contact with others. A period of time may be required where the student is gradually exposed to simple interactions like peek-a-boo, tickling, mild roughhousing, and brief games to increase their eye contact, frequency of approach, and general interest in others. I have found it very important to be "relentlessly fun" with students working on early social skills, frequently playing with them and encouraging others to do the same.

Case Study: Teaching Early Social Interactions

Jack was a three-year-old boy with a diagnosis of autism who made only brief eye contact with others and preferred to isolate himself in a corner of the room away from peers and adults. Usually he manipulated toys in ways that were self-stimulating but not in ways that they were intended to be used. He cried when approached by an adult other than his mother if the adult tried to interact with him for more than a few seconds. He had just started in an ABA program and was at the very beginning of the curriculum when the consultant began a program of teaching social interaction skills by probing Jack's reaction to social events. Approaching Jack during a time of free play, the consultant sat on the floor next to Jack and waited to see if Jack would react to his presence but Jack just continued to spin blocks on the carpet. Sitting right next to Jack, the consultant picked up a block and began to spin it in a way similar to Jack. At that point, Jack grabbed the consultant's block and made an annoyed noise. The consultant gave no reaction and Jack went back to playing. After 30 seconds of quietly sitting, the consultant got up and left.

The consultant waited a few minutes before picking up a small beach ball and calling Jack's name a few times from an area three feet in front of Jack. Jack did not look up or react and continued his manipulation of the blocks. The consultant bounced the ball a few times to attract Jack's attention and Jack briefly looked up. When he did, the consultant threw the ball gently to him. Jack batted away the ball and looked back at the blocks. The consultant retrieved the ball and resumed his original place, calling Jack's name again, this time adding, "Here it comes, it's coming now" in an enthusiastic voice. Jack looked up again and the consultant waited two seconds before launching the ball. During this interval Jack looked up even more and fixed his gaze on the ball in the hand of the consultant. With a huge smile and another "Here it comes" the consultant gently threw the beach ball, which was again batted away by Jack. Following up on the throw, however, the consultant quickly moved towards Jack after the throw and tickled him, saying in a teasing voice, "You can really hit that ball. Why did you hit that ball? Now you'd better go get it." Rather than laugh at being tickled and retrieve the ball to continue, Jack cried and squirmed, and moved away from the consultant.

Similar social initiations were made by the consultant repeatedly over the next few days; sometimes using the beach ball, sometimes attracting Jack's attention with a new musical computer toy, or other novel, interesting objects. The consultant always called Jack's name, enthusiastically talked to him, "invaded" Jack's space frequently but briefly before retreating in order to attract his attention, and ensured that any spontaneous eye-contact or interactive responses of any kind were consequated with additional access to the novel, interesting objects. In addition, gentle pats on the back, brief walking fingers up the arm, and other physical touches were added as consequences. The interactions were brief and the consultant tried to end them on a positive note before Jack protested, but the consultant also tried to gradually require more extensive interaction.

Jack gradually reacted to the social initiation of the consultant by turning towards him more readily and frequently, making brief eye-contact, and sometimes stopping his own play to wait for the consultant to begin. In subtle ways, the criteria for allowing Jack to hold the attractive, novel objects was increased; as soon as the object was brought out and Jack fixed his eye on it, the consultant moved the object around in space at arms length, making noises like "Zoom, zoom." Invariably, Jack would follow the path of the toy for a few seconds before it landed in his lap. Sometimes the consultant would hold the toy on his own head for a few seconds and Jack might look at it briefly while the consultant made a funny face or laughed.

During one session the consultant held up his hand and said, "High five!" and Jack slapped his hand. The consultant then made a series of funny faces, bouncing up and down and emitting strange sounds. For some reason, this greatly amused Jack and he laughed while looking at the consultant. The consultant immediately stopped and held out his hand again, which was promptly slapped again by Jack, requiring a repetition of the "silly" performance by the consultant and with the same effect on Jack. For the third time the consultant moved his hand next to his face and required Jack to look in his eyes for two full seconds. This was easily accomplished as well.

At this point the consultant trained other staff to carry out similar procedures and, over the next few months, Jack's shared attention activities were frequently conducted. After a while he began to initiate contact with others, including the consultant (always looking for a "high five"). Eye-contact, spontaneous approaches, and even simple verbal requests for attention and play increased during the training time. Acceptance and enjoyment of physical contact changed most dramatically. During the training time teaching personnel were encouraged (with the permission of Jack's parents and in a supervised setting) to gradually accustom Jack to tickling, pats on the back, swinging, light roughhousing, and quick hugs. Previously described by some as "tactilely defensive" Jack gradually came to love the contact and it was eventually used as a potent reinforcer for teaching other skills.

Jack's case is not atypical for young students with autism and illustrates the techniques employed for establishing the earliest, most basic social skills. Note that it was important to choose activities that required frequent interactions and provided immediate, enjoyable consequences. As mentioned, the first social games may be brief. *Spontaneous eye-contact* and *approaching others* are principle target behaviors. Other desirable behaviors are spontaneous vocalizations or verbalizations, smiling, physical contact, or requests for play (using gestures or words). The discriminative stimulus or initial prompt for these behaviors is the presence of another person.

Methods of Establishing Early Social Behavior towards Adults

Teaching children to approach adults for fun social interactions may not automatically result in approaches to peers but it is an important first step. Since this training is relatively easy to accomplish and so vitally important it should be part of the curriculum from the very first moment of programming. Social games can be inserted between other curriculum items or made part of a greeting or other brief interaction in passing. They should be done by everyone who interacts with the child often enough to be recognized. Consultants and those who supervise the child's program should recognize that their behavior sets an example for others; they should model spur of the moment, fun interactions with students at every opportunity.

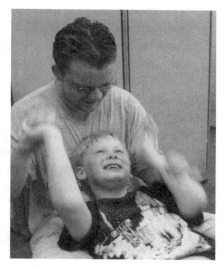

Rather than establishing simple interactions in isolation and then re-teaching them in a more natural setting, it is more effective to begin social training in natural settings (see the discussion on "natural" settings in the previous chapter). The main concern will be to try to promote and reinforce rough approximations of social behaviors at first and then, gradually, withhold reinforcement until closer approximations of the ultimate target behavior are exhibited. Recall that in ABA terminology this is called *shaping*. Shaping requires an effective consequence to reinforce the target behaviors. Consequences intrinsic to social interaction are best if they are effective. It is important for the child to develop an awareness of the intrinsic consequences of social activity because the consequences are naturally and reliably present and do not need to be specially arranged. In other words, students must learn to *enjoy* interacting with others. After they do, the nature of the interaction is often obviously different; there is more sustained eye contact, more spontaneous approaches to others, and it is far easier to teach behaviors that sustain the interaction in interesting, fun ways. But smiles, praise, tickles, funny faces, and roughhousing may not be especially reinforcing for some—at least not at first. It may be necessary to add extrinsic reinforcers like a wind-up musical carousel or even a small amount of a favorite food. If used, extrinsic reinforcers should be paired with social consequences like those listed. Many times after a history of pairing the two, extrinsic reinforcers can be faded.

Timing and choice of target behaviors is most important if shaping is to succeed in eliciting the desired social behavior. The teacher must wait for an approximation of the target behavior, which requires knowledge of how the activity is broken down into component parts. For example, a shared attention activity with a novel toy might be broken down into the following smaller steps:

1. Looking at novel toy
2. Looking from novel toy to adult and back
3. Looking at toy and adult for more sustained periods of time
4. Looking at adult and toy while adult engages with toy briefly
5. Engaging with toy while adult holds (pressing buttons, etc.), and looking back and forth from the toy to the adult
6. Looking at adult when adult approaches with toy
7. Approaching adult when adult enters room with toy
8. Approaching adult and requesting toy when adult enters room without toy

In general the list of behaviors is presented in order of acquisition of the behaviors and later performances include all of the earlier steps. However flexibility in this type of training is important. Shaping is a procedure that requires moment-to-moment judgments on when to reinforce and when to withhold reinforcement. Teachers must be on the alert for the spontaneous appearance of desirable new behavior and remember to require it in later repetitions of the activity.

Even though the teacher must ultimately wait for the appearance of the target behavior in order to reinforce it, various environmental cues and prompts can be used to promote the appearance of reinforce-able behavior. *Proximity* of the teacher is one type of cue, *manipulating an attractive, novel toy* in front of the student is another. When a student has learned to respond well to some of the earlier components of an activity, the teacher may try *pausing* before delivering an expected reinforcer. This may prompt stronger behavior from the student or may provide an appropriate occasion for the teacher to ask for new behavior.

Establishing Early Play Behavior with Peers

While students are learning to engage in simple social exchanges with adults, begin to increase basic peer interactions. At an early stage of play development, the child is likely to have limited skills. Consequently, simple motor activities involving attractive materials are often most successful. Allowing several students to crawl around in a large plastic pool filled with small colored balls (called a *ball bath*) usually provokes many interactions. Assuming that the pool is not too large, the children crawl around, bumping into each other and throwing balls at each other (supervision required!). Often, they emit many sounds (laugh, yell, etc.) which attract the attention and eye-contact of their peers. Several students chasing and kicking a beach ball around an enclosed area also provokes spontaneous interactions including eye-contact, verbalizations directed at each other, and trying to get to the ball first. (It may also elicit less desirable behaviors like pushing, wrestling, and running away with the ball so, again, some supervision is required.)

The success of the activity often lies in the design and choice of materials. Sometimes little things are important. In one game involving throwing a ball over a net in the style of volleyball, no other balls worked as well as large beach balls. Another time when children were chasing bubbles blown by a teacher the size of the room was the key factor. Too small a room and the kids ran into each other; too large a room and they drifted away from the activity. Activities that require close proximity of group members are more likely to promote frequent spontaneous interactions.

It is important that supervising adults not get in the way of participants in the activities. As much as possible, prompts should be minimal in favor of natural consequences from peers. If the activity requires more than minimal prompting it detaches the focus of the child from the peer and pulls the focus onto the adult. Sometimes, however, because of a history of reinforcement for interaction with adults, a particular child will need a certain amount of prompting to get started. In these situations the least level of prompting necessary is recommended starting with what may be called *indirect prompts*. An indirect prompting strategy provides cues to the student without directly using verbal, gestural, or physical guidance. This type of prompting strategy can be demonstrated in an example:

Two four-year-old preschool students, one very inexperienced with interactive play, were seated facing each other in a small sandbox with several toys between them. The inexperienced child had run to the sandbox as soon as he saw the other child sit down and begin to play. However, after being seated, he simply watched the girl play with the sand toys. A paraprofessional assigned to the boy decided that she could intervene to stimulate more interactive play. However, rather than directly prompt the boy to interact with the girl, she followed a more indirect strategy. The paraprofessional sat down in the sand equidistant from both students, forming a triangle with them, and began to energetically play with the toys. She placed a pail between them all and began to fill it with sand saying to the girl with a big smile, "Help me fill this up." When the girl tried to place a shovel full of sand in the pail the paraprofessional "accidentally" knocked the sand off her shovel, saying "whoops" and laughing. (The paraprofessional was careful not to knock the shovel too hard and encourage inappropriate behavior.) Then she announced with exaggerated effect, "I can fill it before you can." At this point the paraprofessional tried to put a shovel full of sand into the pail but the girl knocked the sand off her shovel. Both laughed and began filling their shovels again. Also, the paraprofessional gently tossed an extra shovel into the lap of the boy without further comment or eye-contact; he had been closely observing this rather raucous interaction but made no other movements. The boy picked up the shovel and tried to put sand in the pail too, looking from the girl to the paraprofessional and laughing. After a time the group tired of the game and the girl prompted a replacement, putting a ramp and cars in the middle of the group and pretending to deliver sand to the garage. Spontaneously, the boy took a car and moved it up and down the ramp, sometimes crashing into the truck of the girl. The paraprofessional provided encouraging comments to the group when interest seemed to be waning: "Wow, here comes the truck, beep, beep, beep; crash; there goes the sand..."

The adult never directly prompted the boy to interact with the materials or other players. Rather, she facilitated interaction indirectly by creating a fun, enticing game. Adults can do this kind of prompting in many informal interactive environments like playgrounds, free play in the classroom, snack and lunch, and play time at home. The key elements of this strategy include:

Indirect Prompting Strategies

Choosing simple activities that:
- provide immediate, fun consequences related to interaction
- all of the children can easily perform (often repetitively)

Cheerleading
- Provide enthusiastic encouragement and reactions to actions of the players, injecting a little drama and excitement into the activity
- Try specifically praising the action of another participant doing something that you want the target student to do

Modeling
- If direct participation by the adult is necessary, actually play the game and have tons of fun
- Jump in and out, or fade out as soon as possible

Enlisting Other Participants
- Prompt more experienced players to play in a way that makes it possible for the inexperienced child to easily join in.

Key Skills that Foster Social Interaction and Interactive Play

In the scenarios described above, the students depicted did not engage in complex games or conversations. Social skills develop gradually and, at the most basic level, require very little except an enjoyment of the interaction itself. However, by age three in typically developing children, social interaction and play begins to contain more language and other skills that demand much more from a child with autism. Sample skills that contribute to more advanced interactive play are listed below:

Primary Skills
- Imitating sequences of actions of peers and adults in natural settings
- Following sequences of instructions in natural settings and from a distance
- Knowledge of the names of materials and equipment
- Knowledge of the names of the participants
- Responding to peer's request to play
- Taking turns
- Getting attention from peers and adults

More Advanced Skills
- Approaching peers and asking to play
- Performing movement games
- Performing table games
- Asking for information from peers
- Giving instructions to peers
- Enforcing the rules

The list above is far from complete. Taylor & Jasper (2001) enumerate 61 different programs and Leaf & McEachin (1999) list even more. Melinda Smith, in her excellent and practical book on play, *Teaching Playskills to Children with Autistic Spectrum Disorder* (DRL Books, 2001) suggests that, of all the skills, imitation is the most fundamental skill and the primary vehicle for acquiring social play behaviors. Certainly, mastery of the actual component skills of a particular activity would be prerequisite to doing that activity interactively. For example, if a child is not proficient in rolling and shaping Play Doh, it will be difficult to expect him to engage with a peer in an interactive activity involving making Play Doh foods in a play kitchen. For more material on play activities, including detailed discussions and suggestions of many topics of play see the resource list at the end of the section.

Peer Training

Interacting with peers and groups is made easier for the child with autism if a certain degree of thought is given to the *selection* and *training* of peers who will be enlisted in the interaction program. Selection of peers based on their interaction skills, preferences, or other attributes should depend on the particular activity or situation. For example, rough and tumble gross motor play on the playground requires peers who enjoy such activities while table games, arts and crafts, or computer activities may require different peer participants. Secondly, the social interaction skill level of the peer(s) should be such that the target child has a good model to imitate. The peer model(s) should attract the attention of the target student and promote imitation. This usually occurs if they can competently engage in activities that the target student likes. A student's tendency to imitate a model is linked to the attributes of the model including social status, competence, attractiveness, and similarity of the model to the imitator. For this reason, children that are slightly older than the target student can make good peers, especially if they tend to be naturally inclined to try and please adults by helpfully incorporating the new group member into their play. Some students are inclined to "adopt" other children and actively help them to get involved in activities. They give instructions when the target student seems lost, introduce the target student to their friends, and even prompt other students in the group to be nice to the target student. While this is often extremely helpful, care should be taken that the "helpful" child does not become too bossy or limiting, or begin to feel totally responsible for the welfare of the target student at the expense of their freedom to pursue other activities.

Peers need not be trained teachers and engage in complicated prompting strategies in order to be effective helpers. A few key behaviors seem to be most important:

Key Behaviors for Peers
- Repetition of instructions, when giving instructions to a student who tends to drift from the activity
- Acceptance/ignoring of unusual behavior
- Persistence in social initiations towards the target student even if initially ignored
- Enthusiastic responses to appropriate behavior from the target student

Bridget Taylor, in her chapter *Teaching Peer Social Skills* (2001) summarizes the behavioral literature in this area, enumerating 21 helpful skills for peer assistants, along with a number of effective strategies to teach peers. Often, however, if nurturing children are chosen, their natural interaction style contains some of the behaviors that elicit and/or encourage the right responses from the target student. Subtly and selectively prompting and reinforcing peers *during the activity,* for specific helpful actions can achieve excellent results without pulling children away. It also preserves, as much as possible, the nature of the peer-peer relationship and, perhaps, reduces a loss of social status for the target student. Nevertheless, the complexity of the skills to be taught and the abilities of the target student will dictate the extent of peer training necessary.

Case Study 1

Experiences with prompting peer assistants during interactive play, like the following, lead me to believe that shaping peer skills in place can be highly effective and sometimes preferable to training them prior to the activity or intervention. **Rob**, a seven-year- old boy with autism was fairly new to a 1st grade classroom. His communication skills were rudimentary (single words, a small vocabulary of mands and tacts) but he really loved to interact with the other boys in the room, especially during free-play situations when the activity had competitive components. Prior to Rob joining the class, the teacher explained as matter-of-factly as possible that a new child would be joining them from time to time. She explained that he did not talk very much but that he liked to play with kids his age and that he was learning things just like the other students, even though his work was a little different from theirs. The teacher noted casually that the new student made loud noises from time to time but that they were all going to ignore these sounds and continue with their work. Even though Rob occasionally had mild tantrums including dropping to the floor, it was decided to not include this fact in the discussion with the students but to deal with whatever behaviors occurred calmly with a minimum of reaction and let the class observe (and hopefully imitate) that the teachers were not upset or bothered. It was decided to start Rob's inclusion experience during a spelling lesson (a strength of Rob's) and during the following snack and free play.

One boy in particular, Chris, was very accepting of Rob, and, after an initial suggestion from the teacher, approached him often to play. Chris was a popular, mature boy who was very kind to his friends. Since Rob's interactive play skills were limited, his reactions to social initiations were somewhat unpredictable. If Chris offered to play catch with Rob using bean bags, Rob might ignore Chris until Chris showed him what he wanted to do. Sometimes Chris actually had to physically arrange Rob in place in order to toss him the bean bag. Once begun, Rob enjoyed the interactions enormously, throwing the bean bags to Chris, laughing if Chris missed a catch, and sometimes even intentionally throwing the bag over Chris' head. Over time Chris and Rob learned to enjoy each other's company for many different kinds of activities but a definite introduction period was required for Chris as he learned how to adjust to Rob's unique interaction style.

One day early in the year, Chris approached Rob to play but Rob took no notice and continued to play with a toy truck. Looking a little lost, Chris looked at the paraprofessional assigned to Rob, who was monitoring the situation from about 10 feet away. Without moving, the paraprofessional nodded towards Rob again, smiled at Chris, and mouthed, "Keep going. Get his attention." This time Chris picked up another truck and sat down next to Rob. Twisting around so that he could look directly in Rob's face Chris said, "Let's fill up the dump truck with blocks" and handed Rob a block. Rob began to put blocks in the truck while Chris moved the truck around, dumping the blocks when the truck was full. When Rob saw how the blocks fell to the floor making a noise, he immediately reached for the truck. Chris started to give it to him when the paraprofessional (who had moved closer to the pair) leaned over and said to Chris, "No, keep the truck until he asks for it with words." Chris continued to play with the truck even though Rob made some distressed noises. Finally, he looked Chris in the eye (this time Rob had to twist around) and said, "Want truck, PLEASE!"

Interactions like this continued for brief (5-10 minutes) durations several times per week with 3-4 different children. Gradually they were shaped to interact with Rob in ways that were more successful for all. Initially, specific activities were often suggested for play, based on Rob's mastery and preferences, and on the likelihood that the activity would result in quality interactions. As time went on, less outside structure and prompting was necessary and more free-choice was allowed. The paraprofessional and teacher frequently commented to both Rob and his partners on how well they were playing. Sometimes, after the interaction, the teacher specifically made note of how patient a child might have been or how the child might have been especially clever at showing Rob how to do something. Children were also prompted to include Rob when they played with their other friends. The results were encouraging: after a few weeks, appropriate interactive play in this setting substantially increased. However, it was noted at progress reviews that Rob's language and play skills were holding him back from more advanced types of play. Consequently, specific areas of weakness were identified and worked on in isolation, so that the newly developed skills could be eventually added to interactive play with the group.

Case Study 2

Bill was a six-year-old boy placed in a kindergarten class during snack and recess. On the playground he tended to stay on the periphery of the group. Sometimes he would run around with the other boys, following behind them wherever they would go but not speaking or interacting further. One day, several boys asked the teacher if they could play with Bill on the playground. At first this was puzzling because the boys had free access to Bill and could initiate play at any time. When the boys added, "you know, *really* play" to their request, it became clear to the teacher that the boys were actually asking for adult assistance in making the play more interactive. After giving some thought to the request the teacher chose a large beach ball and asked the boys (including Bill) to join her on the playground.

The teacher chose a simplified soccer activity to introduce to the group but began with a period of probing to determine how best to find a fun activity, one that every participant could do independently, and one that would promote frequent, appropriate interactions. Once in the middle of the field, with the boys clustered around her, she simply threw the beach ball right at one of the boys, gently bouncing it off the top of his head and chasing it herself. The boys did not need a verbal explanation or further invitation. They immediately ran after the ball. Bill stayed where he was. Reaching the ball first the teacher turned around and kicked it back towards Bill. When she neared Bill (with the other boys trailing her) she made sure that the ball rolled right up to Bill and yelled in an urgent voice, "Bill, kick it!" With a herd of young boys running right at him and the ball in front of his foot, Bill quickly kicked the ball in a direction away from the others and laughed. The teacher then yelled, "Quick, quick, get the ball" repeating the phrase as she ran. When she neared Bill she physically prodded him just a bit to get him moving towards the ball. "Run! Get the ball! Who's going to get the ball first?" As Bill started running she slowed her pace, allowing the other boys and Bill to chase the ball and reach it first. At that point the teacher intervened several times to grab the ball and orient it more towards Bill's position. Sometimes she yelled to the group, "It's Bill's turn to kick it," but instructions of that type were rarely necessary because Bill relentlessly chased the ball and, due to his physical prowess, often was able to kick the ball first. The teacher occasionally needed to instruct the boys to move back into the middle of the field. For a while Bill found it funny to grab the ball and kick it over a small fence into a restricted area and it was necessary for the teacher to position herself in front of the fence until he understood that limitation. Mostly the teacher kept yelling encouragement to the boys to keep their excitement level high. She would yell out a sort of play-by-play of what was going on, using one child's name then the other: "Gary's near the ball and here comes Roy. Who will get there first? Ohhhh, it's Roy. Get the ball! Wow, what a kick!" It was especially important to use Bill's name in the same way.

The frequency and quality of interactions during the 20 minutes of this activity were radically improved from previous playground activities. Eye contact with peers was constant, appropriate physical contact was frequent, comments to peers about the activity occurred more than during any other activity, and the interaction was sustained for a period of time longer than was previously thought likely. Judging from the amount of laughing, activity, and noise, the activity was well chosen and well designed. Key elements were:

- **Setting**: the choice of a motor activity on the playground.
- **Equipment**: using a beach ball was a little novel, colorful, and more fun than a soccer ball because it floated high in the air when kicked. It was also safer for the vigorous activity level engaged in by the boys.
- **Simplicity of activity**: running and kicking are straightforward; the element of chasing something added a little competitiveness that worked for this group.
- **Minimal adult prompting**: after getting things started and setting a few limits, the teacher let the kids determine how to play. She strategically intervened to ensure that it remained interactive for Bill.
- **Cheerleading**: Frequent comments from the sidelines added excitement to the activity.

Case Study 3

Casey was a five-year-old girl who loved to play table games, do arts & crafts activities, and engage in imaginative play using dress up materials, play sets, and puppets. During free choice time in her new kindergarten class she could usually be found in one of the play centers devoted to these activities. However, when other children came near she grew quiet and moved to the periphery, turning her back to them and ignoring their attempts to get her to join in. Without any reaction from Casey to reinforce the peers, social initiations decreased sharply. Noticing this, the teacher took aside some of the children who liked to play in these centers and encouraged them to persist in inviting Casey to play. Unfortunately, when the children repeated their invitations and moved around Casey to look at her, Casey moved further away and even covered her eyes.

In contrast to her behavior at school, Casey's parents reported that Casey had no problem playing with her siblings in a variety of play settings, maintaining excellent eye-contact and frequently talking. The teacher decided that Casey needed a more structured experience with her new peers to encourage her to respond to their interaction attempts. Therefore, the next day the teacher arranged for three other girls to play a lively table game with Casey in a quiet corner of the room. The teacher prompted the group to move to the area and set up the game. Casey sat down at the table but looked down, avoiding eye contact with the others until the teacher started talking about her favorite snack:

"Before we start...I gave someone at this table some goldfish crackers and she is going to give some to everybody if you ask nicely." At the mention of goldfish crackers Casey's head came up and she made eye contact with the teacher.

"Ok Allison." The teacher nodded to one of the girls.

Allison, a rather precocious girl, brought out a box and announced dramatically, "Who wants crackers?" just as the teacher had asked her to.

Seeing the crackers, Casey immediately shifted her attention to the box but said nothing until she saw the other two girls asking for and receiving crackers. Quietly but intently following the movements of the girls and crackers for about 15 seconds, she finally reached out her hand and said, "Me too, please," and immediately received about 5 of the small crackers. When she finished these she asked for more without hesitation and received them. After the third round of crackers, the teacher prompted the girls to start the game and put away the crackers. The game chosen was well liked by all of the participants, including Casey, and she quickly became engrossed. She eagerly watched the other girls when they played (even though she did not comment). She carefully took her turn and passed the game equipment when her turn was over. When one girl pulled out the wrong stick and a mass of marbles fell to the table with a clatter, she laughed and clapped, looking at the girls around the table and the teacher.

Several rounds were played with the same result. After about 25 minutes the teacher ended the game and began the next activity with the class. For two weeks the teacher arranged for the same set of girls to play various table games. After a couple of days it was not necessary for her to be in close proximity because the girls, including Casey, played independently, even setting up and cleaning up. The initial snack of crackers was not repeated after the first day. Gradually, the teacher noticed that Casey became more animated and comfortable during the games but she was still reserved and made few comments. One day the teacher talked to Casey just before the start of the game and explained some of the "secret new rules" that would be in effect just for her during the game. The teacher said that she would be watching from across the room and drop a penny into a big glass jar every time Casey said something to the other children. If Casey earned enough pennies she could choose a favorite activity to play with the teacher. The teacher showed Casey the jar and dropped a penny into it, making a distinctive noise that could be heard from across the room. Casey looked at the teacher, smiled broadly, and reacted immediately. "Can we play nurse?" "Yes," said the teacher excitedly. "Let's go start now."

They both walked over to the table and sat down. As they sat the teacher dropped a penny into the jar, looked at Casey, and said, "That one's for free. Remember the rules." The teacher positioned herself about 15 feet across the room so that Casey could easily see her by looking over the shoulder of one of her playmates. Within five seconds, Casey said "Hi" to each girl and heard three pennies drop, one-by-one, into the jar. Then she quickly said hello to the girls a second time which earned the sound of one penny dropping and a mock frown from the teacher that only Casey could see. For the first five minutes of the game the frequency of comments to the other girls was greatly increased from the previous games. After no comments for two minutes the teacher held up a penny and tapped it on the side of the jar. Casey immediately said hello to all of the girls.

While interactions increased using this method, it was also apparent that Casey did not always know what to say to the girls. When more closely questioned about her interactions with siblings Casey's parents confirmed that her range of comments was limited. Therefore, the educational team decided that a speech therapist who was already working with Casey would practice with her some things to say during the games. A list of these phrases was provided to the teacher who gave extra pennies to Casey if she used the phrases.

Discussion of Case Study

The program above first focused on providing Casey with a more structured setting in which to interact. A familiar game was chosen and the other participants were seated in proximity to Casey. The game prompted certain interactions automatically. On the first session an "ice breaker" was included to get things started on a positive note. While successful the new setting was not adequate to prompt many verbal interactions and an extrinsic reinforcement system was added. In addition, specific practice of new verbalizations was done in isolation in order to expand Casey repertoire of things to say. The practice in isolation was specific to the target activity and setting.

Although Casey's program resulted in important behavior changes, several things had yet to be accomplished in the program. First, the extrinsic reinforcement needed to be faded in favor of more natural social consequences. This could have been accomplished once all of the new elements of behavior for the activity had been taught. The team might want to finish teaching Casey more complex ways to talk to the children; new skill acquisition often requires continuous, potent reinforcers. Then, when the new behaviors were strong the extrinsic reinforcement could have been made intermittent and finally eliminated, as long as it was apparent that the natural social consequences would maintain the new behaviors.

Next, using the same peers, new activities (like the original activity centers) could have been introduced. If necessary, the old reinforcer systems could have been re-introduced for a short time. With Casey's previous experience interacting with these girls, generalization of interaction to other, less structured settings may have been enhanced.

Evaluation of Peer Interactions

The choice of methods of evaluation of social interaction and interactive play is similar to measuring participation in other group experiences. The primary challenge is that the settings and behavior is complex. This is alleviated greatly if specific target behaviors are chosen. Once accomplished various characteristics of the behaviors can be measured including frequency of occurrence, duration, number of prompts required, etc. Data collection need not be burdensome but it is essential. One strategy to make data collection manageable is to collect data on a different activity or target behavior each day. In this way each skill is objectively evaluated regularly. For example, Mondays, record the number of social initiations during recess, Tuesdays record the duration of engagement during a tabletop social play activity, and so on throughout the week. (For a list of sample target behaviors with examples of attributes to measure, see the evaluation section of the next chapter.)

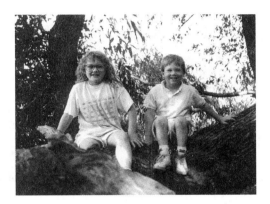

Summary

Social integration and interactive play require component skills just like other skills. Among other things, one must learn to engage in various motor actions, manipulate toys, follow instructions, imitate, and expressively communicate. These skills are gradually acquired and allow the student to interact competently in increasingly complex social situations. Peers may be enlisted and trained to make social activities more successful. Social behavior will probably increase more rapidly if the motivation for interaction is intrinsic to the activity rather than externally delivered. However, reinforcement that is extrinsic to the activity may be necessary for a time to establish and strengthen new behavior.

Key Concepts and Questions

1. What is the difference between *intrinsic* motivation and *extrinsic* motivation in social play?

2. What are some differences between *peer-initiated and structured activities* and *adult-initiated and structured.*

3. What is a common *example* of a peer-initiated and structured activity?

4. Describe an example of a *shared* or *joint-attention* activity.

5. What is *shaping* and how can it be used to increase early social behavior?

6. Describe how *indirect prompts* were used to prompt social play in the example of the children in the sandbox.

7. Name the *key elements* of indirect prompts listed.

8. Name some important skills that contribute to social play.

9. What attributes of peers make them good choices for inclusion in a teaching program?

10. What methods can be used to evaluate programs to teach social play?

References and Resources

Leaf, R. & McEachin, J. (Eds.) (1999). *A Work in Progress.* New York, NY: DRL Books (800) 853-1057; www.drlbooks.com

Smith, Melinda J. (2001). *Teaching Playskills to Children with Autistic Spectrum Disorder.* New York, NY: DRL Books (800) 853-1057; www.drlbooks.com

Taylor, Bridget A. (2001). *Teaching Peer Social Skills to Children with Autism.* In Maurice, C., Green, G., & Foxx, R. M., *Making a Difference.* Austin, TX: Pro-ed (800) 897-3202; www.proedinc.com

Taylor, B. A. & Jasper, S. (2001). *Teaching Programs to Increase Peer Interaction.* In Maurice, C., Green, G., & Foxx, R. M., *Making a Difference.* Austin, TX: Pro-ed (800) 897-3202; www.proedinc.com

Weiss, M. J. & Harris, S. L. (2001). *Reaching Out, Joining In; Teaching Social Skills to Young Children with Autism.* Bethesda, MD: Woodbine House Inc. (800) 843-7323; www.woodbinehouse.com

Chapter 7

GROUP INSTRUCTION AND INCLUSION

Instruction in groups starting in preschool and continuing through the early grades takes many forms—circle activities, arts and crafts, story time, morning meetings, science demonstrations, mathematics games, physical education lessons, and a myriad of other events where students must give their collective attention to the teacher and respond to questions and statements. In preparation for joining such groups the student needs to have mastered a number of basic skills in a more structured and individualized setting (see following section). Also, the student should have participated in small groups of 1-3 other students, practicing interaction with other group members as well as listening to the teacher in a simpler environment. There are many goals for inclusion in larger groups; the most obvious, acquisition of new information, is only one goal of several.

General Objectives for Participation in Group Instruction:

- Increase student's understanding of the complex, natural language involved in multiple sentence presentations and sequences of instructions
- Increase student's ability to follow instructions directed at the group
- Increase student's ability to respond to questions directed at the group
- Increase student's ability to follow basic rules of a group (raise hand, don't interrupt, look at the speaker, etc.)
- Increase student's ability to follow instructions involving performances and materials at a distance
- Increase student's ability to interact with group members about group topic (asking for and giving information, addressing students by name, etc.)
- Acquire information about the topic of group instruction.

Kindergarten is often an entry point for a student's first large, structured group experience. In a typical kindergarten classroom, the teacher leads a group of 10-15 students. Students sit in groups on the floor, at tables, or at desks in front of display boards and tables where the teacher has placed materials for presentation and discussion. The teacher stands 3-5 feet or more away from the group, clearly visible, and in proximity to the materials to be used. The duration of the activities usually ranges from 5 minutes to 30 minutes, but as the year progresses children are expected to actively participate for longer periods of time.

The following is an example of a circle group taken directly from an observation in a kindergarten class during the month of December. The activity was done every day at the same time. The activity is fairly typical for the level of expectations at this time of year. All questions asked by teacher required that students raise their hands before suggesting an answer. The teacher called only on students who raised their hands. (Note that some of the discussion, comments, and transition statements made by the teacher are left out for the sake of space.) The activities are described in the left column and the skills required are noted at the right.

Sample Kindergarten Group Instruction Activity

Description of Activity	Skills Required
1. Teacher softly blows a flute-like whistle and gives an instruction to call students to circle area.. Students interrupt present activity, walk to circle area, and sit on carpet, facing display wall. In order to prompt students to sit cross-legged on the floor, the teacher repeats "Criss-cross, applesauce" a few times.	Following group instructions Following special signals (e.g., "criss-cross, applesauce" meaning to sit down cross-legged on the floor
2. Students talk to each other as they wait for teacher to start. Teacher allows students to mingle for 1-2 minutes, then starts.	Spontaneous language Interaction with peers
3. Teacher: "Good Morning, everyone." Students in group: "Good Morning, Mrs. Smith"	Choral response to greeting
4. Teacher: "Let's start with the news. Does anyone have any news?"	Talking about past and future events
5. Student raises hand, waits to be called on, and states an event that happened or that will happen to him/her. ("I'm going to…" or "I _____ed")	Raising hand before answering. Listening/responding to speaker
6. When finished, the teacher says, "Let's say hello to our friends" and leads the children in a rhyme that greets the students around them. Starts rhyme, "Hey there, neighbor" and students recite rhyme together.	"Choral" recitation of rhymes and songs.
7. Discussion of calendar: Students answer questions on what day, what month, what year, while looking at calendar. Teacher throws in some questions on related things like "What letter does Wednesday start with?"	Wh-questions about calendar. General information questions.
8. Teacher has already highlighted some of the days of the month in a different color so that the days alternate between red and white boxes. The teacher points out the pattern on the chart and asks what kind of pattern it is.	Labeling A-B patterns
9. Teacher starts singing and students follow. Students sing days of the week and months of the year songs.	Choral recitation of Days of Week song and Months of Year song
10. Teacher asks, "What kind of weather is it outside?" Students look outside and suggest answers. Teacher points to words on the chalkboard and students read words aloud together.	Describing weather; Sight-reading in group with materials at a distance
11. Discussion of more/less. Teacher: "Let's count the number of [counters] together." "How many?" "Which one is more? Which is less?"	Counting in a group (choral). Counting objects at a distance. More/less.

12. Reading the schedule. Teacher leads children in reading the things that she has placed on the display board (simple sentences about the things discussed so far in circle like weather, activities, etc.) Children answer questions about what the activities will be during the day.	Sight reading aloud in group Answering questions based on past events.
13. "Can you see a word that begins with "P" on our schedule? Let's count the p's. What p-thing did we do yesterday?"	Following abstract instructions. Recalling past events.
14. Activity preview: Teacher introduces activity materials and asks questions about them. "How many potatoes are in this container? Guess. That's called *estimating*. How many children think that there are 8 potatoes? Raise your hand. Later, when you come back from gym you'll make potato pattern pictures."	Answering Wh questions. Estimating Agreeing/choosing by raising hand.
15. "Now I'm going to read *The Painter*. But first we need to take a break. Ready, everyone stand up." Teacher-aide starts music and students perform the movement game *Head, Shoulders, Knees, and Toes* for one minute singing the song while they do the actions.	Following instruction. Following movement song with actions and singing.
16. Teacher reads story of 8 pages with one sentence to each page. Intersperses questions, explanations,, and comments.	Answering questions based on multi-page story.
End of activity. Duration: 42 minutes	

Many observers are surprised at the complexity of tasks regularly accomplished by kindergarten-age children. The skills required to actively participate in these groups must be specifically taught to some students new to group instruction. Some of the specific skills listed above can be pre-taught at separate, individual times (e.g., the movement song, rhymes, and "criss-cross, applesauce.") Other skills can be reinforced if it becomes apparent that the student needs extra help. Those supervising curriculum development need to observe the activities and the student's involvement regularly in order to help the team target problems and develop the plan of remediation, as we will discuss further below.

> A list of over 100 instructions commonly used on kindergarten worksheets is included in the appendix

Moving from Discrete Trials to a Group Instruction Setting

Obviously, even brief observation in a regular classroom is enough to reveal major differences between the methods of presentation of instructional material in discrete trial formats and group instruction. In any individualized teaching setting the student is expected to wait only inconsequential periods of time, responding frequently to the material. Prompts and the difficulty of material are instantly adjusted to the student's needs, and reinforcers are tailored to the student's tastes. In group situations, the student is often expected to observe other student responses, waiting for a turn to respond. Students need to observe the teacher or speaker as well, respond to instructions given generally to the group by a teacher who is 5-10 feet distant (using materials that are equally distant), respond to complex language with instructions embedded inside several sentences, and to be motivated by intermittent praise or other secondary sources of reinforcement.

When a number of skills have been acquired in a highly structured setting and the team is considering an inclusion setting like a classroom group, a preparation plan should be followed that teaches the student the skills necessary to perform the same mastered drills in a structure increasingly similar to the classroom.

The table on the following page presents a teaching plan that gradually manipulates *five aspects of the teaching setting*.

1. The location of the student
2. The location of the teacher
3. The location and type of presentation of materials
4. The type of prompts used
5. The location of the student performance

For example, imagine that a certain 1st grade student, in discrete trials, has mastered several different forms of imitation, follows instructions well, performs a number of receptive and expressive language tasks, draws or writes figures, letters, and number, and answers wh-questions about pictures and stories.   In Step 1 of the inclusion plan we set up his work area with a student desk and teach him to sit there while performing the drills named above. Gradually, as his performance allows and still using the same drills, the successive steps of the program move the teacher and location of the materials farther away and, then, fade in additional students and more complex instructions. Note that the plan's steps make several changes at once. Some students may benefit from a slower pace with more gradual changes and individual plans should be adapted to the needs of the particular student.

For children in kindergarten or preschool, who do not sit at desks, the sitting location may be changed to a chair, a carpet square on the floor, or a table. The plan should also include specific preparation for unique arrangements of the inclusion group.

Many drills can be conducted during the inclusion preparation process and are necessary for active participation in group instruction. Some are listed at the end of this section. Note that the final target performances should be exhibited *in a group* for all drills.

Combining and Lengthening Performances

Once mastered individually, drills should be combined to form sequences of instructions that the student follows for up to five minutes. In addition, the instructions can be combined so that the student is given two or three instructions before beginning any actions.

Moving from Discrete Trials to an Inclusion Setting
Table: A Sample Teaching Plan
(Bold type indicates changes from the preceding step)

More Structured (1:1)	Step 2	Step 3	Step 4	Step 5	Step 6	Less Structured (typical classroom)
○ Student sits at desk	○ Student sits at desk	○ Student sits at desk	○ Student sits at desk	○ Student sits at desk	○ **Student sits at desk in group of 2 or 3.**	○ **Student sits at desk in group of other students**
○ Teacher sits next to student	○ **Teacher sits 1 foot from desk facing student**	○ **Teacher sits 3 feet from desk facing student, occasionally stands**	○ **Teacher stands or sits 5 feet from desk, facing student.**	○ Teacher stands 5 feet from desk facing student	○ **Teacher stands 5-10 feet from desks facing students**	○ Teacher stands 5-10 feet from desks facing students
○ Teacher presents materials on student desk	○ Teacher presents materials on easel or another table/desk within reach of student	○ Teacher presents materials on easel or another table/desk next to teacher	○ **Teacher presents materials on boards, easels, tables**	○ Teacher presents materials on boards, easels, tables	○ Teacher presents materials on boards, easels, tables	○ Teacher presents materials on boards, easels, tables easily visible by students
○ Teacher prompts with simple verbal and physical prompts, as necessary	○ **Teacher prompts with more complex verbal prompts and gestures**	○ **Teacher prompts with simple, natural language prompts**	○ Teacher uses prompts with simple natural language	○ **Teacher uses natural language instructions directed at group**	○ Teacher uses natural language instructions directed at group	○ **Teacher uses natural language prompts, embeds instructions in multi-part sentences, directed at group**
○ Student makes responses at desk	○ **Student makes occasional responses away from desk**	○ **Student makes responses at desk, while standing, and next to teacher**	○ Student makes responses at desk, while standing, **away from desk,** and next to teacher	○ Student makes responses at desk, while standing, away from desk, and next to teacher	○ Student makes responses at desk, while standing, away from desk, and next to teacher	○ **Student makes responses any place in classroom**

When in-seat instructions are going well, instructions are given to the student that require a performance *away* from the desk. This is often an early component of discrete trial training but must be mastered in each new setting. The teacher asks the student to perform an action away from the desk and then return to his or her desk. The action may involve materials around the room, in the local areas, or at the teacher's desk, table, easel, or board.

Examples:

- o "Count the pumpkins on the felt board" (next to the teacher)
- o "Point to the number 20 on the calendar" (attached to the chalkboard behind teacher)
- o "Get the red book" from the teacher's desk

As the student adapts to the changing circumstances of the location of the teacher and materials, so, too, he or she must become accustomed to the use of more natural language. Simplified language is important for the student when initially learning the meaning of an instruction. However, alternate/equivalent forms of the instruction that vary in wording and length must also be learned. Learning to follow the instruction "Give me ball" needs to be followed by additional training with "Touch ball," "Pick up the ball," and "Please get me the ball." As the student progresses the instructions become longer and more natural sounding. When the student is readily responding to single sentences containing natural language, additional sentences that are not instructions can be inserted:

"*What's this*, Brian? Right, a ball! In fact, there are two balls here—a green one and a blue one. *Point to the blue one.*"

In the example above, the instructions are italicized. Between the two instructions are three statements. The student needs to be listening to each sentence and decide whether it contains an instruction or not. This requires more sustained attention and receptive language skill than simply listening to a single sentence.

When students find themselves in groups, besides the inevitable distractions, they must learn to respond to instructions that are given to the group rather than an individual student. Instead of looking directly at the student and saying, "Bobby, go sit down at your desk" the teacher looks around the room and says, "Everyone, please go sit at your desks." Students need to be specifically taught to respond to group instructions. Following group instructions are especially useful for demonstrating motor tasks to a group, arts & crafts activities, group games, and classroom management.

Following instructions that require a verbal response often involves answering questions. Wh-questions (what, who, where, when, why) and "how" questions are often the heart of teacher-led group presentations. Students need to be able to answer wh- and how questions in order to participate fully in most kindergarten level discussions. Include them as drills when preparing the student for classroom groups. In fact, at the preschool and kindergarten level there are dozens of instructions that involve manipulation of materials, worksheets, books, etc. Refer to the appendix for a list of over one hundred that are commonly used.

Advanced Group Teaching Formats

Group work in a classroom is not a random collection of stories, questions, and worksheets. Instruction is structured so that students become engaged with the topic and master the learning objectives for each activity. The choice of structure of each learning experience is intended to suit the particular learning goals. Several formats or variations are typically seen including:

Demonstrations/explorations: where the students first observe the teacher's actions (usually with accompanying materials), listen to information presented about the activity or materials, and then engage in target activities based on the presentation. Examples: science experiments, arts & crafts.

Presentations: where the teacher gives verbal narratives like stories in which the student listens for an extended period of time and answers questions based on the material presented. Examples: story time, presentation and discussion on specific topics.

Group Interactive Activities: where the teacher leads an activity or discussion in which, primarily, participants take turns engaging in the discussion or activity. Examples: morning meeting, discussing student reactions to current events.

Mixed Activities in which the activity contains a mixture of the above formats, often centering on a theme.

At the kindergarten level, group teaching formats tasks require many skills including asking students to remain in one activity for 15 minutes or more, continuously watch the teacher and/or peers, listen to and understand 2-3 sentences or more before responding, follow group instructions, answer wh-questions (what, who, where, when, why, how), listen to other members of the group and obtain information, imitate the teacher and peers, participate in choral responding, and raise hand/wait turn. If the target student is to actively participate in such groups he or she must have previous experience and some ability in each of these areas.

Description of Formats

A discussion of each format is presented below so that teams may construct learning experiences that allow students to practice the skills necessary to participate in group activities of a similar format.

Format: Demonstrations/Explorations

Examples: Science experiments, arts & crafts, operating a computer, playing a new game.

Description: This format often involves actions with materials or equipment that are usually present and displayed. Students may be seated in a group or even standing (as during a physical education activity). The teacher may display materials on a table, hold them up, or show pictures/movies of the materials. During the display, the teacher talks about the materials in various ways. The teacher may:

- Exhibit and name materials and/or component parts
- Describe/demonstrate features of materials. This includes color, form, size, location, quantity, position, orientation,
- Describe/demonstrate the function of materials. This includes actions (verbs), cause and effect
- Describe/demonstrate operation of materials. This includes actions, sequence, position, orientation

During the activity and after completion the student is often expected to be able to follow multi-step instructions to complete activities involving the topic.

Sequential or Exploratory: The activity may be presented in one of two ways: *sequentially*, with a set order of presentation of information and controlled student input or *exploratory*, with more immediate student engagement with materials and teacher input and questions interlaced throughout. Each sub-format evokes a different set of experiences for the students.

Sample Exploratory Activity

The following activity is adapted from *Sandbox Scientist, Real Science Activities for Little Kids,* by Michael Ross.

Water Droppers (Duration: approximately 15 minutes)

Materials
Plastic water droppers
Large paper clips with one end straightened
Pebbles, erasers, and other objects such as sticks or leaves
Small plastic containers

General Instructions
Place sets of materials on student tables. Fill containers with water. Explain to children why they should not drink the water or poke the droppers in eyes, ears, or nostrils. Show the group the various materials. Ask them to experiment with dripping water on the various objects. Teacher reacts to students' experimentation by encouraging

them to describe what is happening. Students are encouraged to show each other what they have discovered or to copy what others are doing.

Sample Teacher Interactions (only if students need further direction):

- ✦ "What is this called (holds up dropper)?" (Answer: a dropper.)

- ✦ "How do you get water in the dropper?" (Answer: put it in water and squeeze the top)

- ✦ "How can you make the water come out?" (Answer: take the dropper out of the water and squeeze the top)

- ✦ "What happens to the water when you drip it on things?" (Answer: It falls off, it goes inside, it makes the rock wet, etc.)

- ✦ "Make just *one* drop come out of the dropper."

- ✦ "Drip water on the dirty rock. What happens?" (Answer: The dirt comes off.)

- ✦ "Press hard on the dropper. What happens? (Answer: the water comes out faster and goes farther.)

- ✦ "What sound does the water make when it comes out?"

- ✦ "Try squeezing air from the dropper back into the container of water to make bubbles."

- ✦ "Try putting the paper clip into the dropper and squeezing fast. What happens?" (Answer: the paper clip shoots out.)

Discussion of Activity

This activity relies on the natural curiosity of children and their innate tendency to explore. Given the eye droppers and water they may not need much encouragement to engage and interact. However, some children may need a few prompts or guidance. Of course, this guidance should be as minimal as possible since the point of the exercise is to encourage self-initiated exploration. On the language side, children should be encouraged to label what they see if they do not do so spontaneously. This may occur in the form of excited comments to neighboring peers. Without stifling spontaneous commenting, the teacher should try and help students expand their verbal descriptions of what is going on, ask questions about the processes, share information with peers, and discover as many fun and interesting aspects of using droppers and water as possible.

Sample Sequential Demonstration

Arts & Crafts – Making Butterflies (Adapted from "Crafts for Young Children" by Jill Norris). *Please note*: this description is included to illustrate the format of sequential demonstrations. Actual materials for conducting the activity such as templates and step-by-step illustrations are omitted because they are not essential to understanding the organization and structure of the format.

Preparation and General Instructions:

Cover a table with a plastic cloth. Put newspaper on the floor under the painting table. Pour a different color of paint into several flat Styrofoam meat trays and place them in the middle of the activity table. Put a pile of large white paper and colored construction paper in the middle of the table. Next to the piles place a number of 3 inch lengths of string, 4 pieces for each participant, a box of child-safe scissors, a box of pencils, glue sticks, and a box of 6 inch pieces of colored yarn, one for each participant. Construct a template in the shape of a butterfly for each table.

Have students sit at activity tables in groups of no more than 4 children, wearing smocks to protect clothing. Introduce the activity by describing what is going to be done and showing a finished example of the craft. This activity may require some adult assistance.

Sequence of Actions:

1. Take a large white sheet of paper and fold it in half.

2. Unfold the paper and lay it front of you.

3. Dip a piece of string into one color of paint. Make sure it is well coated.

4. Lift the string from the tray and lay it on just the right side of the white paper with the end sticking out over the edge of the paper

5. Do the same thing with several pieces of string dipped in different colors

6. Fold the paper over the strings

7. Press down on the paper with one hand and pull the strings out with the other hand

8. Open the paper and let it dry

9. Fold the paper again. Put the butterfly template so that the straight edge is against the fold and trace around it with a pencil.

10. Cut out the butterfly with scissors.

11. Take a piece of colored paper and lay the butterfly on top of it

12. Glue the butterfly to the paper with the glue sticks

13. Draw a line on the colored paper ½ inch away from the butterfly all the way around.

14. Cut along the line on the colored paper to cut out the butterfly.

15. Punch a hole in the top of the butterfly and thread a piece of yarn into the hole about halfway.

16. Tie a knot in the yarn.

17. Hang the butterfly.

Discussion of Activity

Essentially this activity is a long series of mini-activities involving folding, dipping the strings, tracing, cutting, punching holes, threading yarn, tying yarn, and hanging up the product. The child must follow each instruction in sequence and be able to perform the individual motor actions. The child must perform the actions as part of a group, making his actions and materials correspond to the actions and materials of the teacher or other group members.

Advanced receptive language skills are required involving a large number of individual and combined words and phrases.

- **receptive labels** for each of the materials, actions, and pieces of equipment ("white paper," "colored paper," "string," "paint," "butterfly," "template," "pencil," "scissors," "glue stick," "yarn," "hole," "knot')

- **receptive actions** ("take," "fold," "unfold," "lay," "dip," "lift," "Do the same thing," "press down," "pull out," "open," "cut," "glue," "draw a line," "punch a hole," "thread," "tie")

- **receptive orientation** ("in half," "in front of you," "into," "right side," "with end sticking out," "over the strings," "against," "around," "on top," "away from," "all the way around")

Wherever the child does not understand or misses an instruction she must observe the teacher's demonstration or the actions of a peer. If the child cannot accomplish the task she must ask for help.

Format: Presentations

Examples: Informational topics such as weather, holidays, animals, geography; reading stories aloud.

Description: This format is exemplified when the teacher is the primary presenter of information and the information is primarily verbal. Several sentences or even paragraphs may occur before individual members of the group are given the opportunity to overtly respond. Responses are often prompted by specific questions while spontaneous comments are sometimes ignored as inappropriate. Students indicate willingness to respond by raising their hand and the teacher must distribute the opportunity to respond among all of the participants, thus decreasing any one individual's overt responses. Sometimes verbal responses are choral; other times an individual may be required to leave his seat and interact with materials near the teacher. Students may be seated in groups, tables, or individual desks, depending on the topic. The teacher may:

- Describe events, processes, or read stories
- Describe persons, objects, and actions involved
- Describe features of the topic, including color, form, size, location, quantity, position, orientation, functions
- Describe rules or lessons generalized from the presentation

During the activity and after completion, the student is often expected to be able to expressively name and/or receptively identify certain objects, attributes, functions, and processes involving the topic (what, when, where). Other desired responses may involve cause and effect (why), sequences, compare and contrast (same/different), talking about past events, getting and giving information to the group, and relating relevant personal experiences.

Sample Presentation – Reading a Story

The teacher gathers students in the "Story Corner" by announcing to the group, "It's time for library, boys and girls. Finish up what you are doing and meet me in the Story Corner." The teacher moves to her chair in the area and positions a book on an easel, closed to show the illustration on the cover. The students spend 1-2 minutes gathering in the area, each sitting on an individual carpet square, and talking to their neighbors. The teacher gives a signal to the class to become quiet by rhythmically clapping, a prearranged signal with the class to give their attention to the teacher.

[The teacher picks up the book and points to the cover] Today, boys and girls, we're going to read a story called *The Cat in the Hat* by Dr. Seuss. Does anyone know this story? [She looks around, several children say, "oh" and "yes"] That's great, I'm sure you are all going to like it. It's funny! [Opens book and starts reading first page, finishes page] Look at the way the cat is dressed. What's he wearing? [Everyone calls out, the teacher calls on a girl with her hand raised and the girl says, "A big striped hat"] That's right, Jennifer! But do cats usually wear hats? [Noooo, everyone calls out] Now, everyone, if you want to make a comment or answer a question, remember, raise your hand or I'll have to stop reading. [Turns page and reads the next four pages] What's happening here? Who is the cat? What is he going to do?

Throughout the story the teacher continues to read several pages at a time, stopping to ask various questions of the students. Typical questions include the following and other wh-questions:

- What did he do?
- Why did he do it?
- Why didn't he do that?
- What is that (pointing to an object)?
- Who did that?
- What's wrong with that?
- What is that like?
- Did that ever happen to you?
- What will happen next?

After the story the teacher may review the action by asking students to retell parts of the story and their reaction to it:

"What part did you like best?"

"What did you think when the Cat dropped all of the things he was balancing?"
"Did you ever make a mess like that?"
"How would you like to have to clean up all that mess?"

Additionally, the teacher may try and extrapolate a rule or moral from the story:

"So, should we let strange cats into our house? What about strange people?"

Discussion of Activity

This kind of activity requires sustained attention from participants. The degree of compliance from students (active listening and participation) is usually related to the pacing, number of opportunities to respond, and intrinsic interest of the presentation. However, the degree of difficulty of the language presented (vocabulary, length of sentences, number of sentences per page) is also an important factor. Obviously, simple wh-questions must be mastered in order to participate in the activity. However, student must also become accustomed to more advanced phrasing and questions including questions that are embedded in statements:

"O.K., class, I want you to pay attention to the next few pages because there is something really special in this story. Everybody put on your listening ears and sit up straight. Do you know what a rainbow is? It comes after a rainstorm. Look for the rainbow on this page. *What do you see underneath the rainbow?"* The students' only overt opportunity to respond to the previous statements of the teacher is prompted by the question at the end of the paragraph ("What do you see underneath the rainbow?") However, the students must monitor the *entire* series of sentences for directions in order to respond correctly. Other important skills in this format include

- following multi-page stories read in a group at a distance
- advanced wh-questions (why)
- predicting the outcome
- relating a sequence of events (retelling story)

Variation: Learning about President's Day

In this presentation several activities are centered on the theme of presidents but the responses required from students are still primarily verbal. Students are invited to a section of the classroom where the teacher has set up a large easel with a flannel board, a blackboard, and an auxiliary table with a pile of handouts. With the students gathered together the teacher introduces the activity and hands out a "Weekly Reader" with a picture of Abraham Lincoln and George Washington on the cover.

"Well now, boys and girls, do you know who our president is? The president of the United States?" [Answer: George Bush]. "Yes, that's right, George Bush is our president. He's the president of the United States, of our country. This week we are celebrating President's Day. What's that?" [Answer: the birthday of the president] "Well, yes, that's right. We are celebrating the birthdays of two famous presidents.

Look at your papers. Who can tell me who this is?" [Answer: Abraham Lincoln] "Right! Abraham Lincoln, our 13th president. And, who is this?" [Answer: George Washington.] "Right! George Washington, our 1st president. When were George Washington and Abraham Lincoln the president, now or a long time ago?

The presentation continues by reading a story about Abraham Lincoln and telling a legend about George Washington. Then coins and paper money are passed around to show the students other pictures of Washington and Lincoln, with the teacher pointing to large drawings of the various coins and bills posted on the easel. After 30 minutes the teacher sends the students to their work tables to complete some worksheets related to the presentation. In order to complete the worksheets the students must:

- Match a picture of the presidents (Washington, Lincoln, and Bush) with their printed name
- Complete the sentences, "George Washington was our country's ___ president" and "Abraham Lincoln was our country's ___ president."
- Color the pictures of the presidents
- Circle the date of Washington and Lincoln's birthday on a calendar

Discussion of Activity

Groups vary in their response to this kind of activity. Often a number of children have been previously exposed to the information and eagerly attempt to answer all of the questions while others are silent. For some children there are not enough opportunities to rehearse the information during the presentation and it is often necessary to reinforce key concepts in the presentation with additional questions while students are completing their worksheets. Pre-teaching the material combined with additional practice after the presentation is recommended for students having difficulty.

Format: Group Interaction Activities

Examples: Discussing student reactions to an important current event, planning classroom activities, making group decisions, expressing attitudes and feelings, discussing problem situations, relating past personal events.

Description: In this activity format, the teacher usually guides students into discussing specific questions presented by the teacher. Students take turns speaking on the subject and must remain on topic, addressing the last point (or at least a recent point) made by a speaker. The teacher encourages appropriate verbal behavior exhibited by students through specific reactions, such as reflecting emotions, paraphrasing, and non-verbal behavior such as head nodding and short encouraging comments ("o.k.," "uh-huh," "right," etc) When the conversation lags or gets off topic the teacher intervenes to move the discussion forward.

The student is expected to exhibit several specific skills including:

- Looking at the speaker when listening and looking at the group when speaking

✦ Making statements of personal preferences and opinions
✦ Answering questions involving personal preferences and opinions
✦ Asking clarifying questions of group members
✦ Recalling or inferring information about topics of discussion and/or group members

Sample Group Interactive Activity – Morning Meeting

Morning meetings often take place at the beginning of the day and usually involve a mixture of semi-structured discussion topics, some routine and some new. The purpose of the activity is sometimes described as "preparing" students for the schedule of the day, "processing" occurrences or events, or "sharing" with the group. Specific activities contained within a morning meeting vary considerably, but examples include talking about the past weekend's activities, recognizing birthdays and special individual events, show-and-tell, talking about problems within the group, talking about upcoming field trips, and talking about the day's schedule.

The teacher begins the morning meeting by giving an instruction to the group to move to a specific area of the classroom. The group often sits on the floor or in chairs, close together, in a semi-circle around the teacher so that each student can see all members of the group. The teacher greets the group and introduces the first topic:

"Hello and good morning everyone. I hope you had a good weekend. What are some special things that you did on Saturday or Sunday?" Children raise their hands and the teacher calls on one student. The group listens to the student relate a story about a visit from his grandparents over the weekend and where they went to have fun. The teacher uses open-ended questions to help the student expand the descriptions of the events and use as many descriptors and full sentences as possible. The teacher then invites other children to react and ask questions. Some spontaneous comments or questions are tolerated but teacher reminds the students to raise their hands to ask questions. The student speaker calls on other students and answers their questions for 4-5 minutes. At times, the teacher intervenes to ask the group for a reaction to a certain aspect of the student's presentation like, "Did you ever go on a picnic like Danny and his family?" After the allotted time is up, the teacher moves on to the next student. Four students present in this way before the teacher transitions into the next topic.

"You all sound like you had a great weekend. Now we need to discuss what we are going to do today. Remember that Mrs. Bean is going to come in and help us do our cooking. We are going to follow a recipe and make pudding just before snack. [Teacher puts a small sign that says *Cooking* on the schedule board.] But before that, since it's Monday, we're going to the library. Did you remember to bring in your books from last week?" [Teacher puts *Library* sign on schedule board. The teacher continues describing the day's coming events until all of the time slots are filled—about 8 different activities. She dismisses children from the group by telling them to line up for library according to tables.] "O.K., table 3 first on line; now, table 1; table 2; table 4."

Discussion of Activity

Full participation in this activity requires more advanced conversational skills such as describing past events, asking and answering questions about student presentations, and observing and attending to others in the group. Fairly sophisticated receptive language skills are a must. Students must be able to separate out instructions and key bits of information that are embedded in multiple sentences, a sometimes difficult task when the operative parts of sentences are surrounded by a great deal of verbiage that is extraneous to the activity. First of all, the student must be familiar with prefaces to sentences like "O.K., now, I want you to…" and other natural language fillers and expressions that populate common speech. Secondly, students should practice following longer *sequences* of instructions expressed in natural language. Gradually, the complexity and variety of language and required responses can be increased as the student learns to stay with the activity and be more fully engaged for longer periods of time.

Since verbal responses in a group are usually made one participant at a time, opportunities to respond for an included student may need to be manipulated, initially, in order to provide adequate reinforcement to establish a strong, consistent performance. The student may need to specifically practice turn taking and attending to other speakers in a simulated group where the frequency of being called on is gradually thinned to levels seen in the classroom. Once in the classroom a transition period may be necessary during which the teacher calls on the included student more frequently.

A good curriculum will provide an enumeration of many of the skills important to functioning in group interactive activities; see the curriculum areas of **conversation-advanced, asking questions, peer interactions, and social awareness** in *A Work in Progress* by Ron Leaf and John McEachin (DRL Books, 1999) or the chapter, *Teaching Programs to Increase Peer Interaction* by Bridget Taylor and Suzanne Jasper in *Making a Difference* (Pro-Ed, 2001).

Evaluation

As with all interventions that attempt to change behavior, evaluation of the results of inclusion experiences and group instruction can occur in many ways but *regular data-based assessment of specific target behaviors* should be the centerpiece of the evaluation. While some on the educational team may fear that data collection would be difficult or burdensome, it need not be. Especially at the outset of inclusion, when the student is first practicing new skills in a group setting, additional personnel should be available to ensure that the important details of acquisition receive proper attention. Prompts need to be strategically delivered and carefully faded, and reinforcement needs to be tailored to specific learning situations. In order to properly evaluate the results of instruction and provide a basis for any needed revisions of the methodology, objective data collection on individual target behaviors is indispensable. Here again, classroom support personnel can perform a crucial duty.

Enumeration of specific target behaviors must be part of setting up the individual goals and programs of the curriculum. The methods of evaluation should also be specified. The following table lists some common target behaviors for group instruction activities along with some methods of evaluation

Sample Target Behaviors	Possible Evaluation Method(s)
Follows signal to assemble in correct location for group	Occurrence/nonoccurrence
Brings/obtains required materials	Occurrence/nonoccurrence
Engages in appropriate social behavior while waiting	# of social initiations and responses
Looks at speaker	Duration; percentage of time
Follows instructions	Percent correct actions; complexity/content of instructions; list instructions are *not* followed
Responds to questions from teacher	Percent correct answers; length of answers; vocabulary used; latency of response
Responds to questions from other students	Percent correct response; length of response; vocabulary used; latency of response
Asks questions	Frequency; content of question
Imitates other students	Frequency
Raises hand to answer	Frequency
Makes spontaneous comments related to activity	Frequency
Completes activity	Frequency; number of steps; number of prompts required; description of actions completed

Understanding the methodology of evaluation is straightforward, especially for those who have already conducted behaviorally-based programs in other settings. However, actual implementation of a consistent data collection system in the classroom and adherence to data-based decision making must not be thought of as superfluous. While challenging at times, it rewards implementers with a level of understanding of the student's status that is unequaled without it. Nonetheless, several things can be done to make the task of data collection easier. Data sheets can be based on schedules so that a minimal amount of page flipping is required. Target behaviors can be defined so that a simple check suffices to record occurrence. In addition, *samples* of activities can be taken; that is, data on a particular activity can be taken once or twice a week rather than every day, or data can be taken for a short period of time that is representative of the whole activity. Abridged or abbreviated methods of data collection are not problematic as long as the method arranged provides a reliable and valid picture of the student.

DESIGNING AN APPROPRIATE INCLUSION EXPERIENCE

The decision to have a student spend all or part of the program day in a typical classroom, with typical, same-age peers, is one charged with hopes and expectations. Parents rightfully expect their children to be placed in the "least restrictive" learning environment possible—hopefully, one that is the same as other children who may not have a diagnosis. Unfortunately, the process of making such a decision can be, sometimes, more reflective of wishful thinking on the part of the educational team—the "place and hope" strategy of program creation—rather than a result of an honest assessment of the child's abilities in the critical areas of classroom and group functioning. It is crucial to adequately prepare for inclusion and address the key determinants of its success.

Key Factors in Successful Inclusion

Generally, a successful inclusion experience is more likely to occur when:

⊕ the student has some basic prerequisite skills

⊕ the student's time in the classroom is carefully planned, addresses specific goals, and progress is measured objectively and frequently

⊕ the student is accompanied full-time by a familiar individual who has a strong history of successful teaching with the student

⊕ individual time outside of the classroom is used to support classroom skill development

⊕ the program is closely supervised by personnel experienced in ABA and there is access to a senior-level ABA clinician

⊕ the educational team thinks of inclusion as a process rather than an all-or-nothing program

The aim of a student spending time in a classroom or other inclusion experience with other students is that the student learns while interacting with others, acquiring social experiences, skills, relationships, etc. The degree to which the student already interacts with others is an important factor in determining the amount of time spent in groups and the nature of the inclusion experience. The student's time is valuable; a balance must be sought between the amounts of time spent in concentrated individual work vs. inclusion time. Nevertheless, an inclusion experience can often achieve educational goals unattainable elsewhere, providing a new and stimulating environment for the child.

The following are helpful skills for classroom "survival" at the preschool or kindergarten level but they are not strictly prerequisite. Many students have some of the skills but lack others. This should not be a problem if the child is ready to pick up the skills that he or she lacks. It should be emphasized that, even if a number of skills are not present in a student, there may be substantial benefit to spending time in a typical classroom. The extent of likely benefit can only be properly judged on a case-by-case basis by an educational team that knows the student well and follows the principles of specific, goal-directed planning and objective measurement of progress, discussed above.

Skills That Contribute to a Successful Inclusion Experience

General

- Looks at speaker
- Waits in line, waits quietly for activity to begin
- Refrains from stereotypic behavior in public
- Toilet trained (self-initiates)
- Listens to multi-page story for 3-5 minutes
- Raises hand before answering
- Sits with group in different classroom locations for up to 20 minutes (on floor, at desk, at table).
- Manipulates arts and crafts materials including drawing, painting, scissors, clay, coloring, glue, etc.

Following Instructions

- Follows instructions in a group
- Follows instructions when teacher is across room
- Follows conditional instructions
- Follows multi-step or sequenced instructions

Imitation

- Imitates behavior of others spontaneously
- Imitates sequence of actions
- Imitates in a group

Matching

- Identical object-to-object and picture-to-picture matching of objects, colors, shapes
- Non-identical matching
- Associations (sock-foot, glove-hand)
- Sorts into categories
- Letters, 3-4 letter words
- Complex matching (two attributes such as object name and color-blue bear- or object name and size-big car)

Language

- Responds to greeting and initiates greetings
- Receptively identifies and expressively names objects, actions, attributes, functions, and categories found in classroom as well as in books.
- Spontaneously asks for desired/needed objects
- Asks for help
- Answers wh-questions based on story
- Prepositions
- Answers basic personal questions (what's your name, how old are you, etc.)
- Sings songs with group
- Describes past events

Academic
   * Rote Counts to 20
   * Counts objects to 20
Play
   * Watches others play/approaches
   * Seeks others to play
   * Responds to others play initiations
   * Plays appropriately with a variety of equipment present in classroom
   * Plays independently for 20 minutes
   * Plays movement games in group
   * Plays simple board games/takes turns/follows directions

Goal Setting and Evaluation for Inclusion

Sometimes programs that carefully and objectively document student progress for individual programs in an isolated setting are surprisingly lax about doing the same for programs occurring in the classroom, as if, upon entering the classroom, one crosses the threshold of a new and different world where altogether different learning principles reign. The classroom may have an unfamiliar organization, new students, sights, sounds, activities, rules, etc., and there is a consequent temptation to abandon the methods that have successfully brought the student this far in their learning career. Obviously, this temptation must be resisted. Nevertheless, the complexity of the classroom environment does offer challenges to goal setting and evaluation as well as implementation of programs.

Proper planning is the most powerful tool in tackling these challenges. Working together with the classroom teacher, the educational team should identify appropriate settings and activities, and set specific goals for the student in each setting. Successful participation and completion of an activity must be task-analyzed (broken down into small component parts) and a strategy to teach the activity to the student devised, including prompts, reinforcement, and any other necessary teaching components, *including data collection procedures*. This process is repeated for *all of the activities* in which the student participates in the classroom. Care should be taken to evaluate all aspects of the student's inclusion experience. The curriculum should specify these specific goals and, in addition to academic performance, usually includes goals for social interactions, language, play, and independent functioning *in group settings*.

Data collection is the primary means of evaluating the student's progress but observation and verbal reports of teaching personnel can also be helpful in providing information on progress. In addition, an experienced ABA clinician should observe the student as often as possible to obtain a source of information not dependent on others.

Using Individualized Time to Support Inclusion

After just a few days in a typical classroom many needs of the student that were unforeseen will be glaringly apparent. The team needs to plan to meet soon after the student starts in order to deal with these issues. Some planned activities will be found to be inappropriate or unworkable while others will be extremely successful. Adjustments in goals, procedures, and activities will result in a better plan for the student.

Depending on the skill level of the student, it is usually necessary to arrange supportive instruction *away from the classroom*, in a less distracting, more individualized environment. For example, if a child does not seem to understand many of the questions of a story because the story is read too rapidly for him, the instructional assistant might read the story with the student *before the group story time* and go over a few wh-questions. With the added practice, the student might more confidently respond to the same story during the subsequent group story time. Many variations of *pre-teaching* are possible; some pre-teaching activities can even occur *in* the classroom.

Individualized time is usually required for quite some time after the student begins an inclusion experience. In addition to pre-teaching, a myriad of more advanced language, academic, and even components of play and social skills often require introduction in distraction-free environment before integration into the group, so that a smoother, more errorless performance is obtained. The reinforcement that follows more successful participation in the group may motivate the student to try hard, both in individual practice and during the group time, and eventually need less teaching in isolation.

Checklist for Inclusion Planning and Preparation

Here's a checklist of ideas, hints and advice regarding inclusion:

✦ **Prepare for inclusion**
  - Teach as many preparatory skills as possible, like those mentioned under "Skills That Contribute to a Successful Inclusion Experience" above
  - Teach in small groups as often as possible
  - Try "reverse inclusion" (bring 1-3 volunteer students from the classroom into the student's program areas for play, games, or other fun activities)

✦ **Use the student's strengths and interests as a guide on where to start**
  - Does the student plays well with others? Start at recess
  - Does the student likes stories? Start at story time.
  - Does the student like music, gross motor activities, or a specific teacher? Start with an appropriate corresponding activity

✦ **Establish excellent instructional control in different settings**
  - The student should follow directions immediately, even in distracting situations or when absorbed in a favorite task
  - Do group instruction drills in the target classroom *when it is empty*

- Develop a "remote control" prompting strategy (that is, an unobtrusive way of communicating with the student from a distance. This is especially helpful for prompting during social situations)

Identify a teacher and class that will be receptive to the student.

- The student is not a guest! He or she must become a full member of the classroom community. It is up to the team to help the student find an appropriate role and be accepted in the group based on his unique personality, skills, and goals.

- While the student is in the classroom, the classroom teacher is the student's teacher, not the paraprofessional or the special education teacher. The support team is vital in assisting the classroom teacher to help the student achieve his or her place in the classroom but that will not happen unless the classroom teacher has the same role for the included student as for the typical students.

Make sure the classroom teacher is part of the student's educational team and fully discuss history, characteristics, and goals of the student with the teacher. Include the classroom teacher in trainings on applied behavior analysis and solicit his or her input at meetings

Consider discussing the arrival of the student with the class *before* the child attends. Weigh the benefit of preparing the class for possible unusual behavior against the risk of calling unfavorable attention to the new student. Consider asking a few mature students to occasionally pair up with the new student and help him or her feel at home. Train the students to overlook behavior problems such as yelling and to be persistent in social initiations towards the new student.

Summary

More than anything, inclusion and instruction in groups requires educational team members to understand the specific components of the target curriculum and group settings enough to adequately prepare the student. Careful planning, preparation, and close teamwork are vital components of a successful program. The foregoing presentation of activities is illustrative of the types of activities seen in a typical early inclusion experience and will help as a guide in curriculum development. However, careful attention to each unique activity in the target group will be necessary in order to design an individual plan for each student.

Key Concepts and Questions

1. Name two general objectives for students participating in group instruction.

2. Observe a group activity in a regular preschool or kindergarten and list specific skills required to participate.

3. List the *five aspects of the teaching setting* discussed in the chapter and describe how they are manipulated to help a student move from an individualized, discrete trial setting to group instruction.

4. Design and conduct an activity similar to the type described in the chapter as a *demonstration/exploration*. Include a list of prerequisite and target skills for the activity.

5. Design and conduct an activity similar to the type described in the chapter as a *presentation*. Include a list of basic skills required for participation in the activity.

6. State a convenient way to collect data on the target skills listed in the two questions above.

7. Name several key factors mentioned that contribute to a successful inclusion experience.

8. Name several skills that are important in an inclusion experience.

References and Resources

Norris, J. (1997). *Crafts for Young Children.* Monterey, CA: Evan-Moor Educational Publishers. www.evan-moor.com.

Ross, M. (1995). *Sandbox Scientist, Real Science Activities for Little Kids.* Chicago IL: Chicago Review Press, Inc.

Part III: Planning the Student's Curriculum

The actual process of constructing an educational program has several steps:

+ Evaluation of the student and determining a baseline performance
+ Implementing the first draft of a comprehensive program
+ Evaluation of progress and revision of the comprehensive program

Chapter 8

ORGANIZING AN INDIVIDUALIZED CURRICULUM

OVERVIEW

A student's educational program consists of a set of programs addressing goals in several developmental areas, determined by the educational team to be necessary at that particular time for the student to achieve the optimal degree of independent functioning.

Program Domains

The curriculum must address the child's needs in a variety of developmental areas called *domains*, including at least:

- Language and Communication
- Social Interaction
- Play
- Gross and Fine Motor
- Cognitive/Pre-academic/Academic
- Self-care and Independent Living
- Community Involvement
- Behavior

Settings

All of these skills are addressed, ultimately, in each of three settings: *home, school, and community*. For example, language must occur at home, at school, and in the community, albeit in different ways. Specific self-care activities vary from setting to setting but occur in all three. Academic skills like reading and writing are important in all aspects of the student's life as well.

EVALUATION OF THE STUDENT

Assessment of a child is accomplished in a variety of ways including diagnostic evaluations, health-related examinations like neurological and audiological testing, formal intelligence tests, behavioral, communication, and family assessments, physical and occupational therapy evaluations, and curriculum-based measures (1999, NYS

Department of Health Clinical Practice Guidelines). A comprehensive program is multi-faceted and requires information from a wide variety of sources. The educational team must sift through this information and specify an appropriate set of initial target skills, basically answering the question, "What should be taught and in what order?" For this purpose there is nothing more helpful than a comprehensive curriculum-based assessment. Curriculum assessments are based on a developmentally sequenced list of critical skills attained by typical children in the target age range, and categorized by skill domains and sub-domains. For example, the Autism Partnership curriculum (Leaf & McEachin, 1999) covers skills from birth through kindergarten and lists over 50 curriculum areas with over 500 individual skills. The *Individualized Goal Selection Curriculum* (Romanczyk, Lockshin, and Matey, 1996) lists 19 curriculum areas, each further broken down into levels, stages, and tasks (over 2000 tasks in all).

Initial assessments using developmentally sequenced skill lists with a broad scope provide a specific and detailed picture of the student's current skill level that helps formulate the initial curriculum; a curriculum-based assessment forms the core around which the program is organized. In the following sections a system of developing an individualized curriculum from the assessment phase through implementation and revision is presented. The system uses forms and organizes an individual student curriculum with the aid of a special software program (*The Consultant's Companion*) included on the accompanying CD-ROM, greatly speeding up the process and eliminating and automating much necessary but tedious paperwork. The set of goals included with the software are used for the examples that follow but the methodology is not specific to a particular curriculum. Any comprehensive set of goals may be used. Blank copies of the forms illustrated are included in the appendix and on the CD if you choose not to use the computer software. The specific organizational procedures and forms presented have been used for three years in a center-based program for young children with autism and represent a simplified approach to organizing programs. Simplicity in organization combined with a certain amount of zeal in program housekeeping seems to result in the best managed and most consistent programs. Creativity and spontaneity may contribute mightily to programs but organization and management keep them going. Straightforward and less complicated organizational strategies are more likely to be implemented and maintained, leaving the educational team (and especially the teachers) more time to work with students. The first section presents information on completing a curriculum-based assessment called the *Curriculum Worksheet*. (Please note: if you have not yet obtained a curriculum, several resources are listed at the end of this chapter.)

The Curriculum Worksheet—Determining a Baseline Performance

Those who know the student best are in a good position to communicate information about the student's skills and problems. A list of the curriculum's target skills in all areas of development, called a *curriculum worksheet* is presented to those knowledgeable about the student such as parents or former teachers. Depending on the curriculum, this list may be included in a special evaluation section or it may be necessary to provide a working copy of the entire curriculum to the informant.

Informants read each target skill description and mark the item according to the level of mastery of the student. The following code has been used in the present system:

   ⊕ **(NR): Not Ready** – The student is not ready to work on the item/has no prerequisite skills

   ⊕ **(C): Current** – The student is currently working on the area and has some ability *or* the student *could* work on the item.

   ⊕ **(M): Mastered** – The student has mastered the item

If data exists related to the item the informant is encouraged to provide a summary. If not, the informant is encouraged to choose a performance level based on their best *personal* observations and recollection. If they have not observed performance of a particular skill, informants write "no information." If the informant is completely unsure about a particular item, a question mark is entered instead of the codes. Those filling out the assessment are encouraged to give their best estimate but to not spend more than 15-20 seconds on each item. Explanations, comments, or other additional information pertaining to the items are written in the margins or on the back of the checklist sheets. Usually, informants are given a few days to one week for completing the curriculum assessment

At this time, three additional informational forms are filled out by the informants. The *Student Information Form* contains information that is vital for every person working with the student to know, including special dietary information, medications, special medical conditions and allergies, fears, contact information, permissions, and any other important information. Since it is seen by the entire team, private information is not included here.

The *Potential Reinforcers* list is a place where informants can write down a student's favorite foods, drinks, activities, toys, events, interactions, etc. This information will provide a helpful starting point for identifying reinforcers.

> ⊕ A copy of these forms is included in the appendix.

The *Mand List* is a list of known opportunities to ask for things that occur on a regular basis throughout the student's day. To a great extent this intersects with the child's interests, wants, and needs. The mand list is an attempt to begin to document the times when the child will be required to use language to obtain certain things. See the section *Organize a Mand List* in the chapter on language training for more information.

Probing the Curriculum Worksheet

Once the worksheet is complete a consultant or experienced program coordinator reviews the material, looking for items that have been marked as mastered or partially learned. These items are listed according to curriculum area on a *Probe Data Sheet* and given to those who will begin to systematically present the student with the activities listed on the Probe Data Sheet. Mastered and partially mastered items are chosen because, at this stage, data-based procedures provide the most reliable information, and confirmation of mastery or non-mastery is required to identify the goals that will be the most appropriate candidates for inclusion in the initial curriculum.

The choice of items to probe requires some judgment and a few decisions. It is relatively easy for students with few existing skills but much more time-consuming for advanced students. In the case of beginning students the initial steps of the basic programs will be probed. For students who have mastered many skills in many curriculum areas it would be inefficient to probe *all* mastered items. Instead it is suggested that, for each curriculum area, probes include just one or two mastered skills that *precede* non-mastered skills. If it is subsequently found that those mastered skills are not, in fact, mastered, earlier skills can always be probed. For an example of deciding which curriculum items to probe, see the table below. Imagine that the area of *imitation* is being probed and that the curriculum breaks the steps or sub-skills in this curriculum area into the following:

Curriculum Worksheet					
Goal Number	Curriculum Area	Step	Specific Area	Goal	Mastery
44.00	Imitation	1	Imitation with Objects	Student imitates actions with objects.	M
45.00	Imitation	2	Motor Actions	Student imitates gross and fine motor actions involving head, arms, hands, fingers, legs, feet, trunk, whole body	M
46.00	Imitation	3	Oral-Motor	Student imitates movements involving tongue, lips, and teeth.	C
47.00	Imitation	4	Imitations in a Series	Student imitates series of up to 10 actions with single initial verbal cue "Do this." Teacher waits to model next action until student imitates present action.	C
48.00	Imitation	5	Crossing Midline	Student imitates actions involving crossing midline of body, e.g., touching left knee with right hand.	M
49.00	Imitation	6	Out of Seat and Return	Student imitates actions with or without objects, going to location, doing imitation, and returning to chair	C
50.00	Imitation	7	Imitating Others	Student imitates person indicated by teacher.	M
51.00	Imitation	8	Two-Step Sequence	Student imitates two-step actions where teacher models both actions before student begins.	NR
52.00	Imitation	9	Three-Step Sequence	Student imitates three-step actions where teacher models all actions before student begins.	NR
53.00	Imitation	10	Imitates Action in Freeze-Frame Video	Student imitates action in video immediately after model performs action if video action is "frozen."	NR
54.00	Imitation	11	Imitates Action in Photo	Student imitates action given in photo given instruction," Do that."	NR

The student's mother has provided the estimates of mastery in the right column. Note that the student is marked as not ready (NR) to work on the more advanced imitation skills in steps 8-11. The first two steps are consecutively mastered but the middle steps are mixed between mastered and current. In this case, since the imitation drills are relatively easy to present, it may be wise to put steps 1-7 on the probe data sheet and probe all of them several times over a period of time. On the other hand, in probing step 4 (imitations in a series) imitations with objects, gross and fine motor imitations, oral-motor imitations, and crossing the midline may all be included in the sequence of actions modeled. If the person probing includes all of these actions in the stimulus list, it may be possible to get the necessary information on all of the drills in question at once.

It should be emphasized that information gained from the probes is preliminary. It is not unexpected that students in new and unfamiliar circumstances and working with new teachers may not perform at previous levels. This does not necessarily mean that reported previous performances are in error or that the performance is lost. The child may be temporarily failing to generalize and may rapidly improve once they become accustomed to the new surroundings, materials, and personnel. Nevertheless, it is important to establish what the new student will do in the specific new teaching environment and begin at the level indicated by the student's performance in that environment. If the probe data underestimates or overestimates the "real" ability level it will become readily apparent as teaching continues. Adjustments are expected and easily made in these initial phases of individual curriculum development.

In order to complete the Probe Data Sheets, personnel must be familiar with the methodology for conducting the particular skill program associated with the listed goal performance. Curriculums should have a step-by-step skill program that is associated with each goal, used to conduct the probes but methodologies from other sources or specially written may be preferred. The team member coordinating completion of the probe data sheets must make sure that those actually conducting the probes are trained in all of the skill programs associated with the probes.

A software program called The Consultant's Companion that organizes student information and creates this form is included on the CD-ROM. A blank copy of this form is also included in the appendix

Data Sheet   Page 1 of 8

Current Programs for: John Student
Setting: Drill

I - Independent
P - Prompted
C - Spontaneous

Curriculum Area	Item:	Description:	Date and Data:
Comprehension	1 What?	Student answers what questions based on pictures or story.	
Social Awareness	16 Table Games	Student will play simple table games, following rules, taking turns, and manipulating pieces (e.g., Uno, Candyland, Chutes and Ladders, Connect Four, War, Bingo, Memory, Don't Break the Ice, etc.)	
Recall	1 Actions	Student names action just performed.	

31-Jul-01 9:37:33 AM

Probe items are presented multiple times so that data can be collected on student performance and so that personnel can actually observe the student performing the target skills. The activities are presented in different settings whenever feasible so that the extent of generalization can also be determined. Detailed information on performance is also recorded on the reverse side of the form concerning the level of performance of the student (e.g., the specific items named, actions imitated, instructions followed, etc.) Together, the *Curriculum Worksheet* and the *Probe Data Sheets* comprise the *baseline performance* of the student on the curriculum.

The First Draft of the Curriculum

Once the baseline is established, the needs of the student are prioritized and the educational team decides what drills and activities are most necessary to work on first. The initial *individualized curriculum* is drafted for the student, shown in the example below.

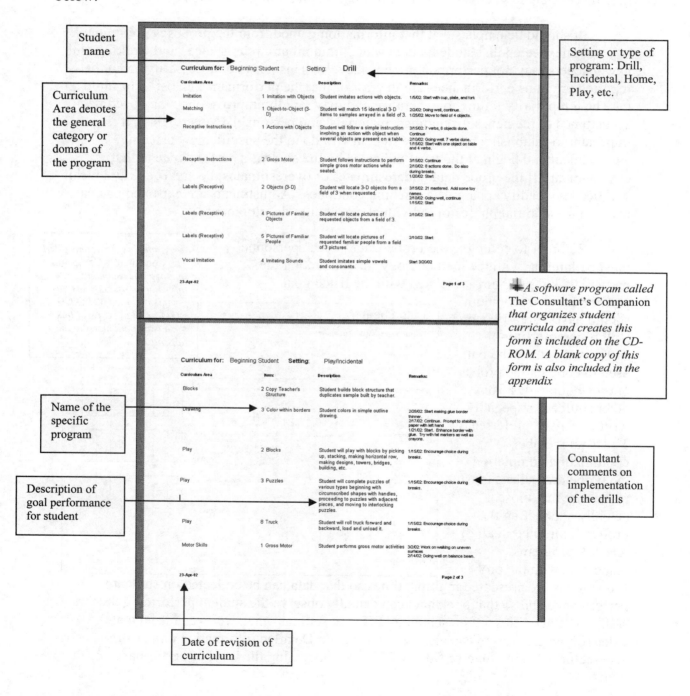

Format of the Individualized Student Curriculum

The individualized student curriculum is intended to supply day-to-day guidance to implementers. Ostensibly, it is a list of skills to be worked on organized according to curriculum area. However, this list offers a central place for including other important information. One piece of helpful information is to include review comments on each specific item. When performance on a curriculum item is reviewed by the consultant, coordinator, or teacher, changes in implementation or student status may occur and may be noted. Dated documentation of ongoing implementation efforts can be summarized next to the curriculum item easily with the use of a word processor or the software program included. It is also helpful to sort the curriculum list by *setting* as well as curriculum area. When a team of implementers works with a student it is important to be clear about *where* the focus of implementation should be. Some skills are implemented at school, some at home, some on the playground, and some at lunch. Some are implemented in all settings. Any meaningful location or setting name can be chosen:

- Teaching formats ("discrete trials," "incidental," "play")

- Activities ("break," "lunch," "morning meeting")

- Locations ("cubby," "cafeteria," "classroom," "playground," "home," "all")

- Times ("morning," "Saturday")

Factors Influencing Choice of Initial Target Skills

Educational research on sequence and scope in skill development has produced inventories of skill development referenced to typical child development (e.g., Brigance, 1978), and can be very helpful in getting an overall sense of normal skill acquisition. Target skills for every student must be age appropriate as well as functional and it is crucial for the educational team to have a realistic picture of what skills are required at a particular age. This will help avoid presenting a student with tasks that are too difficult, do not fit well into the peer group, or take valuable time away from more useful subjects. For example, the development of social play, imitation, and spontaneous requesting is crucial at the earliest ages, even though these are extremely difficult for many students with autism and PDD. Since skills in these areas are acquired by many typical children *prior* to preschool, such programs for students already in preschool or older should receive priority in their curriculum and should not be displaced by other target skills. Sometimes this occurs when a child is particularly strong in a certain area and there is a temptation to go forward in an area of relative strength. While there is nothing wrong with this reasoning per se, care should be taken to ensure that enough resources are devoted to the acquisition of the most age-appropriate and functional skills.

Another reason that typical age-referenced skill inventories cannot offer more than general guidance to the educational team is that each child is different in their learning style, history, motivations, strengths, and deficits. This corresponds to a unique path of acquisition for each particular child even if their more general course is typical. For example, although receptive language tends to be acquired before expressive language in typical children, I have observed that the reverse has been true for some early expressive language tasks with some autistic students. It seems that the students in question were strong at echoing a verbal model and learned to name an object before identifying it when asked to point to the object. In addition to resulting from a strength, the "out of order" performance may also have been related to a weakness in the students' ability to listen and receptively match auditory stimuli with the objects

Finally, many early learning skills develop in parallel once the so-called "learning to learn" skills develop. Acquisition of skills such as eye-contact, joint attention activities, requesting desired items, simple gross and fine motor skills, motor imitation, identical matching, following simple instructions, identifying common objects and familiar people, and imitating sounds and words, seems to open up a number of parallel paths of skill development that intersect at various points and diverge at others. Further skill acquisition continues by adding to and extending existing skills. Gradually, new curriculum areas and settings become relevant. Of course, curriculum items are not learned in isolation from each other. Skills in one setting must be generalized to other settings, teachers, and natural language instructions. The curriculum must specify when and where this is to occur. The ultimate question for each curriculum item concerns its relevance and contribution to achieving the immediate and long-term goals of the student. The clearer the rationale for including each particular item, the easier the educational plan will be to evaluate, maintain, implement, and eventually achieve.

Continuous Evaluation and Revision

At frequent meetings between the consultant and educational team there is a revision of the student's individualized curriculum according to the progress made. These reviews often drive the pace of progress, providing specific target dates for implementers to strive towards and are very important. Participation must include parents and paraprofessionals. I find that four hours per month divided into two 2-hour blocks every two weeks is the minimum acceptable time allotment for curriculum review, with additional time necessary in the beginning. Some students require much more time. Objective criteria for mastery of each educational activity are set as part of each skill program and, at these meetings, the student's performance is compared to the established criteria. Implementation methods are reviewed to help ensure that the most successful procedures are being employed and problems or issues related to program implementation are raised. Minutes of the discussion and a revised copy of the curriculum is then printed out and stored in the program book.

The person responsible for specifying the curriculum is also responsible for directly observing and working with the paraprofessional and student in order to evaluate student progress. As part of the monthly time allotted above, the consultant or experienced coordinator observes and participates in implementation of the student's curriculum, offering corrections and advice on methodology, answering questions, brainstorming solutions to problems, and modeling new techniques. Periodically more structured feedback should be given in the form of an objective evaluation like the *Teaching Evaluation Checklist* or *Program Audit* (see appendix). Program reviews and observations can also be used for on-the-job training of personnel and parents. See also the chapter *Required Competencies for Instructional Assistants* under the "Ongoing Training" sections. With some programs, especially center or school-based programs, in addition to the consultant, a person with some advanced training in running ABA programs is usually available on a daily basis to directly supervise implementation. This person may be a certified special education teacher with training in ABA, a "lead therapist," a "program coordinator" or other individual who oversees and supports the day-to-day operation of the program and consults with the paraprofessionals when problems are encountered or when students advance. This can be a real advantage and is recommended whenever feasible.

All of the items that are mastered by the student are tracked according to their date of mastery. A list of such drills, called the "Mastered List" is kept in the program book.

Advanced Student: Mastered List

Goal Number	Curriculum Area	Phase #	Specific Area	Goal	Mastered
12	Non-verbal Imitation	8	Two-Step Chains	Student imitates two-step actions	11/24/1999
13	Non-verbal Imitation	9	Crossing Over	Student imitates actions involving crossing midline of body, e.g., touching left knee with right hand.	11/24/1999
10	Non-verbal Imitation	6	Continuous Chain	Student imitates series of actions with single initial verbal cue.	11/24/1999
9	Non-verbal Imitation	5	Fine Motor Imitation	Student imitates 17 fine motor actions	11/24/1999
7	Non-verbal Imitation	3	Imitations Away From Chair	Student imitates 14 actions with or without objects, going to location, doing imitation, and returning to chair	11/24/1999
6	Non-verbal Imitation	2	Large Motor Actions	Student imitates 18 gross motor actions.	11/24/1999
5	Non-verbal Imitation	1	Object Manipulation	Student imitates 30 actions with objects.	11/24/1999
14	Non-verbal Imitation	10	Two Responses at Once	Student imitates two actions given at the same time.	11/24/1999
17	Non-verbal Imitation	13	Imitates Action in Photo	Student imitates action given in photo.	1/14/2000
8	Non-verbal Imitation	4	Imitates Another Person	Student imitates person indicated by teacher.	2/11/2000
11	Non-verbal Imitation	7	Advanced Imitation	Student imitates actions involving fine distinctions such as raising one vs. two arms.	9/15/2000
681	Non-verbal Imitation	12	Imitates Action in Video	Student imitates action in video: single action, two-step action, three-step action, continuous chain of actions, two-step delayed action, three-step delayed action.	1/8/2001
18	Block Imitation	1	Building a Tower	Student builds a tower in response to verbal direction, eight blocks tall.	1/14/2000
19	Block Imitation	2	Discriminates Colored Shapes	Student matches seven different blocks varying by shape and color to identical sample in a field of three.	1/28/2000
20	Block Imitation	3	Sequential Steps	Student constructs block design by imitating teacher's actions, step-by-step, in all possible block placements (on top, left vs. right, front vs. back, orientation of block).	2/11/2000

Tuesday, August 28, 2001   *Page 1 of 15*

The mastered list addresses the need for documentation of progress and provides ongoing feedback on the student's pace of acquisition. It can be useful at administrative reviews of student progress (i.e., IEP reviews) where the allocation of resources is discussed, as evidence of the efficacy of the student program or need for further resources. A more clinical use of the mastered list is to use it as a basis for generalization, mixing drills, and developing additional curricula.

CREATING AND MAINTAINING A STUDENT SCHEDULE

A student's curriculum can get fairly complex and implementation must be organized so that the activities of all members of the team can be monitored and coordinated. There are several ways to do this but one important way is to create and maintain a student schedule. The schedule lists the major activities done throughout the day on a regular basis and has many benefits including:

- Organization of all components of the student's curriculum so that the proper frequency of implementation can be planned

- Components can be arranged according to the most beneficial order and time of day

- Frequency of completion of schedule components can be monitored for individual components as well as overall numbers of components

Constructing a Schedule

The initial student schedule is constructed after the baseline assessment by the student's team including consultants, teacher, parents, paraprofessionals, and additional service providers. A draft is drawn up by the team at the first clinic, with input from any additional service providers. Thereafter, the schedule is completed and maintained daily by the paraprofessional under the supervision of the certified teacher, lead therapist, or program coordinator. At program meetings it is helpful to review past schedules in order to determine whether the program is being implemented aggressively enough or if there are any schedule problems, including an imbalance in the number of times programs are implemented or conflicts in scheduling.

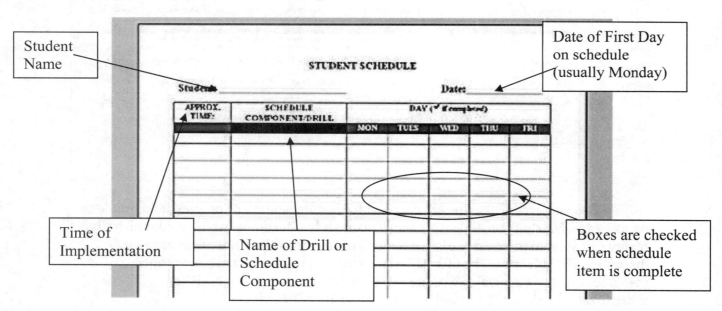

A sample blank schedule form is shown above. The form is started at the beginning of each week when the paraprofessional writes down all of the major scheduled items in order of their implementation. Items that are done more than once are repeated. Items that are *not* done every day are still written in the order of their implementation. If a second sheet is necessary it is attached. Comments can be written on the back of the sheet but should be dated.

Change is Inevitable – (Don't Worry, Be Happy)

Approximate times are written for each item but these times are not usually expected to represent *exact* times. The schedule is created for the student, not the other way around; it is a planning aid and, as such, represents only an estimate of what actually occurs. The paraprofessional is responsible for adapting the schedule to the needs of the student at any given time. For example, sometimes drills may last longer than expected. Sometimes it is appropriate to repeat a new drill on a given day several times. Other times a child may be having a difficult day and certain activities may be shortened or others substituted. In these cases the actual activity that occurred is written in the appropriate check boxes (with, possibly, a notation on the back of the sheet).

Once again it is important to emphasize that changes to the schedule are inevitable and expected in a good program. Occasional changes and adaptations should not lead, however, to a chaotic or unpredictable day. Even when some activities are changed the overall shape of the day should be consistent.

Breaks? – Not in the Schedule

In a manner of speaking there *are no breaks in a schedule*. By this we mean that the student is considered to be *always* in a program during the times covered by the schedule and, therefore, the schedule should have no gaps. Certainly this does not mean that drills are presented to the student every moment. The schedule needs to be created with various activities including lunch, snack, recess, indoor play, and free-choice time as well as drills and more "academic" sounding things. There should be no such thing as "down time" in the sense of a time when there is no stated plan of what is supposed to happen and what our responsibilities, as teachers, are to the student.

If the child is awake each moment presents learning opportunities that must be seized. While this may be intense for teacher personnel, it should not be so for the student. From the student's point of view, the series of events in his or her day should be well-paced, fun, and interesting, allowing for occasional, natural periods of quieter, more sedate activities or (with very young children) even naps. There should be an ebb and flow to the day's events—exciting, challenging activities that are completed interactively can be alternated with quieter, more solitary activities. This does *not* mean, however, that the quieter, more solitary activities are breaks for the teacher. Teachers should ensure that the child has constructive activities available during *every moment* of the day.

Incidental Teaching and Generalization in the Schedule

Seizing on every minute of the day and capitalizing on as many learning opportunities as possible is the ultimate goal for the student's team. The combination of activities on the schedule combined with a philosophy of making every moment count will multiply the amount of teaching well beyond the minutes spent at a table. *Incidental teaching* has been discussed in an earlier chapter and can be very powerful. For example, if, during a "break" in the presentation of a series of discrete trial drills, the child is allowed to choose from among a number of play items (puzzles, picture books, dolls, trucks, blocks, etc.) a number of learning opportunities present themselves. In addition to the skills acquired from playing with the toys themselves, teaching personnel can ask the child questions, set the occasion for eye contact and shared play, give directions, and reinforce spontaneous verbalizations.

The schedule should include items that are specifically planned for natural environment times (play, social interaction, gross motor activities, self-help skills, etc). Using the mastered list to promote generalization, teaching personnel present short opportunities for students to engage in mastered drills in various locations throughout the day. Sometimes it is helpful to set aside a longer period of time, one or two times per day to work on randomly chosen, mixed sets of trials from the mastered list. For example, after snack the child may remain at the table with the instructor. The instructor may then ask the student to touch a few body parts, identify some objects in the room, follow an instruction or two, or perform some other actions from the mastered list. These mixed drills are especially good for children who tend not to listen carefully to instructions and rely on repeating the performance that was reinforced on the last trial.

Incidental teaching and generalization efforts are extremely important and must be included in the schedule. Efforts to use incidental teaching times and mixing mastered drills should be evaluated on a regular basis as part of the formal observation process (see the *Teaching Evaluation Checklist*).

Summary

A student schedule aids in the organization and implementation of the student's curriculum and makes that implementation something that can be reviewed and revised. Schedules need to account for *all* of the student's time in the program and should be created keeping in mind the student's need for diversity and consistency. Implementing a good schedule involves understanding how to capitalize on the learning opportunities involved in *all* of the schedule components, not just the drills.

SETTING UP THE PROGRAM BOOK

Each student should have a three-ring binder dedicated to containing all of the program materials—program write-ups, lists, data sheets, etc. Usually, a two-inch binder is necessary and sufficient. Sections are created with dividers for each of the programs on which the student works. In addition, sections are created for the various lists that are helpful, notes of meetings, and the current curriculum (program list). A sample set-up might look like this:

Program Book Sections

Section	Description
Section 1	General Information (quick facts) on student including medical alerts or allergies.
Section 2	Student's Schedule
Section 3	Language Programs: Mand List, Word Lists, other language instruction materials
Section 4	Potential Reinforcer List
Section 5	Curriculum (Current Program List)
Section 6	Behavior Program (if applicable)
Additional Sections	A separate section for each curriculum area containing: Individual Programs/Drills. Each program section includes: - Program Write-Up - Stimulus Lists - Data Sheets - Graphs
Section	Mastered Drills
Section	Meeting Minutes

(*Helpful hint*: individual sections for each curriculum area may be organized so that the data sheets and stimulus list pages directly face each other, making easier the process of positioning the book conveniently to take data during drills. This is accomplished by punching holes on the right side of the data sheets and on the left side of the stimulus lists. For left handed instructors, the reverse may be more convenient.)

Additional books or files will be needed to contain the initial baseline evaluation and probes, old program write-ups, data sheets, stimulus lists, and graphs, etc. A communication book may also be helpful in communicating informally between educational team members including teaching personnel and parents.

Key Concepts and Questions

1. List the domains important in establishing a comprehensive curriculum for a young child with autism or PDD.

2. What three settings should be addressed by any curriculum?

3. Referring to a curriculum, what does *sequence and scope* mean?

4. What are some sources of information in a comprehensive evaluation of a student?

5. What is a curriculum-based assessment?

6. In the present system, what two processes comprise the baseline evaluation?

7. Where does information for the Curriculum Worksheet come from?

8. Discuss how to decide what items from the Curriculum Worksheet should be included on the Probe Data Sheet.

9. How is the individualized curriculum organized in the present system? Name the features and format.

10. What are some limitations of strictly following normal development in choosing curriculum for a student?

11. Discuss the recommendations for evaluation in the present system including the content of program review meetings.

12. How is the Mastered List used in the present system?

13. What is meant by "there are no breaks in a student schedule?"

14. Name the sections of the program book. How are the sections on curriculum areas arranged?

References and Resources

Brigance, A. H. (1978). *Brigance Diagnostic Inventory of Early Development.* North Billerica, MA: Curriculum Associates.

Leaf, R. & McEachin, J. (Eds.) (1999). *A Work in Progress.* New York, NY: DRL Books (800) 853-1057; www.drlbooks.com

NYS Department of Health, Early Education Program (1999). *Clinical Practice Guideline, Report of the Recommendations. Autism/Pervasive Developmental Disorders.* Albany, NY: NYS Education Services. P.O. Box 7126, Albany, NY 12224. (518) 439-7286.

Romanczyk, R. G., Lockshin, S. & Matey, L. (1996). *Individualized Goal Selection Curriculum.* Apalachin, NY: Clinical Behavior Therapy Associates, Suite 5, 3 Tioga Boulevard, Apalachin, NY 13732, (607) 625-4438.

Sundberg, M. L. & Partington, J. W. (1998). Teaching Language to Children with Autism or Other Developmental Disabilities. Pleasant Hill, CA: Behavior Analysts, Inc. 3329 Vincent Road, Pleasant Hill, CA 94526

Part IV: Training and Evaluation

Foremost among the necessary items in our arsenal for program creation are found the topics of staff training and program evaluation. Both are central in effective, well developed educational programs. Part IV contains two chapters presenting:

1. A training curriculum for establishing primary skills for personnel working directly with students.
2. A tool for assessing the overall effectiveness of an ABA program

Chapter 9

SUGGESTED COMPETENCIES FOR PARAPROFESSIONALS

Personnel who work individually with students may not have specific prior training in behavior analysis, special needs, or autism, although it is mostly through the quality of their efforts that students will achieve their educational objectives. In turn, the quality of their efforts is directly related to the training received. At the present time no national certification is available that is specific to working in ABA programs with autistic children and there are few dedicated training programs. However, in the area of general behavior analysis, entrance to a certification exam is available for those with a 4-year college degree, six months of supervised experience, and 90 classroom hours of training in applied behavior analysis. Successful completion of the exam results in certification as a Board Certified Associate Behavior Analyst™.

While prior training and experience is fervently sought after in paraprofessionals, the state of the field at the present time usually requires extensive training of new staff. This poses a recruitment and training challenge to programs desiring to serve new students, requiring the establishment of effective staff training resources and dedication of ongoing resources. The training materials below represent the *minimum* level of competency suggested in the various performance areas *prior* to or soon after beginning work with a student. Skills designated with a ✦ are the most critical and basic while skills designated with a ✦ may be acquired in subsequent training. Note that the word *orientation* designates target performances in the trainee that are primarily verbal and descriptive, as in being able to name the phases of a discrete trial. The word *implementing* (as in "*implementing* a language program") designates target performances in the trainee that are applied, in the sense of implementing the steps of learned procedures with students. In the present set of competencies, verbal performances are evaluated through questions while applied performances are evaluated through observation.

Specific Duties

Paraprofessionals are responsible for directly implementing educational programs with children. They generally work individually with a child but may also work with their student in a group, depending on the program. Instructional assistants usually work under the direct supervision of a certified special education teacher or lead therapist and the general supervision of a qualified ABA consultant or program coordinator. Specifically, they are responsible for organizing and presenting the educational tasks and materials, prompting behavior when required, and reinforcing or correcting behavior.

They must be familiar with the specific curriculum areas and drills relevant to their student as well as general teaching and behavior change techniques.

Paraprofessionals must be able to evaluate the student's performance and communicate the results orally and in writing. In conjunction with the educational team as a whole, the paraprofessional creates a daily schedule of activities from the curriculum prescription developed by the consultant and implements it with the child, adjusting when necessary. Under the supervision of the certified teacher, lead therapist, or consultant, the paraprofessional decides when a specific performance criterion has been achieved and when to move the student to the next prescribed program step.

The paraprofessional is an important member of the student's educational team and communicates both formally and informally at meetings and in other settings with the parents, teacher, consultant, and administrators.

Summary of Competency Topics

- Orientation to Autism/PDD

- Orientation to Applied Behavior Analysis and ABA Programs for Children with Autism

- Basic Principles of Learning

- Teaching Formats, and Settings (orientation and implementation): discrete trial, generalization, incidental, social play, language, group instruction

- Orientation to the Individualized Student Curriculum

- Implementing the Student's Daily Schedule

Training Title: Orientation to Autism/PDD

Purpose

The purpose of this training is to develop the verbal behavior of trainees with respect to causes and the nature of autism and pervasive developmental disorder so that they can better participate in discussions concerning their student that involve remediation of various aspects of the disorders.

Target Skills

After attending this training, trainees will be able to:

- Describe autism and PDD-NOS as:

    - Conditions appearing in children before the age of 3 years
    - Labels belonging to a general condition called Pervasive Developmental Disorder

- State the words signified by PDD-NOS.

- Describe three attributes of autism or PDD-NOS.

- State one difference between autism and PDD-NOS

- State, yes or no, whether mental retardation is always a component of autism and PDD-NOS.

Ongoing Training

- Identify attributes of the trainee's student that fit their diagnosis and which attributes are not present.

Reference

American Psychiatric Association, Diagnostic and Statistical Manual, 4th Edition, section on *Pervasive Developmental Disorders*.

Training Title: Orientation to Applied Behavior Analysis and ABA Programs for Children with Autism

Purpose

The purpose of this training is to help trainees learn to talk about the field of applied behavior analysis and primary principles of learning, discriminate ABA in general from ABA programs for young children with autism, enumerate the features of ABA programs for young children with autism, and discuss the efficacy of ABA methodology.

Target Skills

After attending this training, trainees will be able to:

- State what ABA stands for and explain the significance of each word in the designation.

- State several fields of concern for applied behavior analysis

- State the results of Lovaas's 1987 study.

- State several requirements of "ABA" programs for young children with autism that are identified with effective treatment.

- Discriminate between descriptions of behavior that are observable and objective and those that are not.

- Why does the scientific study of behavior require that behavior be defined in observable and objective terms? What's wrong with mentalistic descriptions of behavior like, "He was happy all day."

- State the components of the Behavioral Timeline.

- What are contingencies?

- Name four kinds of contingencies or consequence-based procedures.

- Define each consequence-based procedure with respect to *operation* and *function*. Provide an example of each involving students with autism.

- Name some limitations of *sole* use of reinforcers and punishers.

- Discuss how to keep students engaged. Include the concepts of pacing and presentation, and opportunities to respond.

- Discuss the importance of individualization, novelty, and satiation in choosing reinforcers.

- Evaluate a particular teaching environment and discuss ways to eliminate distractions.

- Using the same environment chosen above, discuss ways to arrange it differently so that learning is better facilitated.

- How can choice be incorporated for students who do not directly communicate choices.

- What is a task analysis? How is it used in errorless teaching?

- Task analyze the skill of riding a bicycle.

- Why are mistakes counterproductive to learning?

- What is functional analysis?

- Name two general reasons why behavior occurs.

- Why intervene early with problem behaviors?

References

Maurice, Green, & Luce (1996), *Behavioral Intervention for Young Children with Autism*. Chapter 3, *Early Behavioral Intervention for Autism: what does research tell us?* by Gina Green.

Chapters 1 and 2 of *The ABA Program Companion*.

Ongoing Training

- Read "Let Me Hear Your Voice"
- Read other articles on efficacy of various treatments for autism

Training Title: Orientation to Discrete Trial Teaching

Purpose

The purpose of this training is to teach trainees to identify and discuss the components of discrete trial teaching in preparation for performing the steps with their students.

Prerequisite Topics

Introduction to Autism
Efficacy of ABA
Overview of ABA
Observing and Describing Behavior
The A-B-C's of Behavior Analysis
Proactive Steps to Teaching (Using antecedents)

Target Skills

After attending this training, trainees will be able to:

- Define the word *discrete* as used in discrete trials

- Name the 4 events of a trial

- Name 3 important concepts in *Obtaining the Student's Attention*:

  - Set up the environment beforehand

  - Wait for attention; attract attention only if absolutely necessary

  - Keep student's attention with fast pacing and short inter-trial interval times

- Name important concepts in *Present the Instruction or Prompt*

  - Each skill program has an instruction associated with it that is designed to evoke a response from the student

  - The instruction can be any stimulus: a word, sentence, signal, presentation of object.

  - Instruction gradually comes to control the response from the student and is then called a discriminative stimulus

- Name important concepts in *Student Responds*

  - A specific, objectively defined target behavior is designated correct for each trial

- Name important concepts in *Deliver Consequence*

  - Potent reinforcer is delivered immediately with praise for correct performance.

  - Reinforcers must be strong

* In some cases an error correction procedure is delivered for an incorrect response

⊕ Name 3 prerequisite skills for Expressively Naming Colors

⊕ Fill in the blank: "Breaking skills into component parts and moving forward in small steps forms the basis for an (*errorless*) technique of teaching."

⊕ Why are errors to be avoided?

⊕ Errorless teaching focuses on which event in the sequence of *4 events of a trial* presented earlier?

⊕ *Stimulus Control* refers to control of what? (Behavior)

⊕ What stimuli are referred to in *Stimulus Control* (Stimuli that come before the behavior)

⊕ Name one way of ensuring a correct performance using stimulus control.

⊕ Name several steps of a prompt fading strategy for physical prompts.

⊕ What is a *most-to-least* prompt fading strategy?

⊕ Using the manual, name five dimensions of antecedent helping stimuli that can be changed to fade out their use.

⊕ What is the definition of *free responding*?

⊕ Without referring to notes, state the steps of the generic error correction procedure.

⊕ What happens if the student still responds incorrectly after several error correction trials?

⊕ When is free responding used?

⊕ Without referring to notes, state the steps of the generic discrete trials teaching procedure. Define *massed practice, random rotation with prompts,* and *random rotation.*

⊕ What does *practice in isolation* mean?

⊕ With the instructor or another trainee serving as student and using the stimulus list included with the drill, demonstrate 10 trials of one of the five sample programs. Then, add a new performance and demonstrate another 10 trials. Include in the demonstration fading out the helping stimulus. Do not take data.

⊕ Give an example of a simple discrimination and a conditional discrimination.

Reference

Chapter 3: Teaching in Discrete Trials, *The ABA Program Companion*

Training Title: Implementing Discrete Trials

Purpose

The purpose of this training is to teach trainees to present instructional materials and learning opportunities to students using correct, fluid, and rapid technique.

Target Skills

After attending this training, trainees will be able to:

Given a drill with several stimuli in random rotation:

- Describe how a given drill should be performed
- Choose an appropriate time in the daily schedule to conduct the drill
- State the stimuli that have already been mastered and those that are presently being taught
- Demonstrate how to arrange stimuli and materials including seating of the child, position of the instructor, arraying the stimuli for each trial, readying the reinforcer, and positioning additional stimuli.
- Demonstrate how to attract the attention and eye contact of the child including requiring proper student seating.
- Demonstrate the proper moment to present a learning trial.
- Demonstrate good technique in delivering reinforcer.
- Demonstrate optimal pacing of learning trials.
- Demonstrate immediate recording of data after each learning trial.
- Provide the least effective level of assistance to the student as needed.
- Provide error correction procedures according to drill specifications.

With the instructor or another trainee serving as student and using the stimulus list included with the drill:

- Demonstrate 10 trials of all five sample programs included in Chapter 3. Then, add a new performance and demonstrate another 10 trials. Include in the demonstration fading out the helping stimulus. Fill out a stimulus list and data sheet for the program. Take data during the demonstration.
- With a student who has mastered all five programs, demonstrate each of the programs and receive feedback from an experienced observer based on the Teaching Evaluation Checklist.
- Calculate student performance and graph.

Training Title: Implementing Discrete Trials (Continued)

Ongoing Training

- Practice different techniques for attracting and keeping the students attention
- Refine pacing and presentation of learning trials
- Refine error correction techniques and prompting.

Reference

Chapter 3: Teaching in Discrete Trials, *The ABA Program Companion*

Training Title: Mixed Drills, Generalization, and Incidental Teaching (Orientation and Implementation)

Purpose

The purpose of this training is to teach trainees to implement mixed drills and incidental teaching techniques according to stated specifications.

Target Skills

<u>After completing this training the trainee will be able to:</u>

- Name three kinds of generalization and discuss why generalization is important?

- Identify where to document generalization on the stimulus list form.

- State the purpose of mixing drills.
- Give two reasons for teaching incidentally.

- Give an example related to the following statement: while teaching in a natural environment may be one example of incidental teaching, incidental teaching may also occur during structured teaching.

- Give an example of a primary activity and skills incidental to that activity.

- State how reinforcement could be "captured or contrived?"

- Describe the logic behind organizing incidental teaching according to setting or activity.

- Demonstrate mixing drills in a discrete trial setting and incidentally.

- Demonstrate contriving a reinforcer in order to require language during a play activity.

References

Chapter 3: Teaching in Discrete Trials, Chapter 5: Incidental Teaching, *The ABA Program Companion*.

Training Title: The Language Program—Orientation and Implementation

Purpose

The purpose of this training is to teach trainees to implement an ongoing, all-day program of language instruction based on the curriculum specified by the consultant and teacher.

Target Skills

After completing this training, trainees will be able to:

- Define the terms *mand, tact, intraverbal.*

- Give an example of receptive and expressive language.

- State, when modeling or prompting verbalizations, what should be modeled and what should not be modeled.

- Describe a *mand list* and state why one should create a mand list.

- Define the term *communication temptations* and provide examples.

- Describe how to teach mands.

- State how often language training should occur.

- Name some *individual components* of the language curriculum that might be taught in isolation first.

- Give two examples of *sentence stems.*

- State why language drills are mixed after they are mastered separately.

- Define RFFC.

- Name the seven basic elements of a sentence, according to Larsson.

- Give an example of a two-term sentence using Action/Object.

- Give an example of a three-term sentence using Subject/Action/Object.

- Give an example of reciprocation performance where a student responds to a statement with another statement.

- Explain the following statement: "In order to teach students to ask questions, the environment should be arranged so that asking questions becomes necessary, frequent, and functional."

With their individual student:

- Model new verbalizations to student in a correct manner

- Follow the student's mand list

- Follow the student's tact list (if existent).

⊕ Identify new, appropriate words for tacts and mands

⊕ During a 30 minute observation, exhibit proper techniques for encouraging language in a natural setting including, contriving reinforcers, reinforcing spontaneous verbalizations, proper prompt usage and fading, appropriately requiring elaborated language, and inclusion of appropriate skills.

References

Chapter 4: Components of Language Training, Chapter 5: Incidental Teaching, *The ABA Program Companion.*

Training Title: Social Interaction and Integration

Purpose
The purpose of this training is to teach trainees to effectively promote social interactions in natural settings using the least intrusive prompting strategy possible.

Target Skills
After completing this training the trainee will be able to:

Answer the following questions:

- What is the difference between *intrinsic* motivation and *extrinsic* motivation in social play?

- What are some differences between *peer-initiated and structured activities* and *adult-initiated and structured*.

- What is a common *example* of a peer-initiated and structured activity?

- Describe an example of a *shared* or *joint-attention* activity.

- Name the listed steps in the shared attention example with the novel toy.

- What is *shaping* and how can it be used to increase early social behavior? Explain how you would use shaping to gradually teach the steps listed in question 5. What important things did the consultant do in this example?

- Describe how *indirect prompts* were used to prompt social play in the example of the children in the sandbox.

- Name the *key elements* listed.

- Name some important skills that contribute to social play.

- What attributes of peers make them good choices for inclusion in a teaching program?

- What methods can be used to evaluate programs to teach social play?

Given an available group of typical peers and a student that is the target for social instruction:

- Design a simple activity to encourage interactive play

- State the target behaviors for the student with autism

- Exhibit effective indirect strategies of prompting as often as possible

- Use the least intrusive direct prompts required and exhibit proper fading

- Exhibit effective, momentary peer instruction methods during the activity.

Reference

Chapter 6: Social Interaction and Integration, *The ABA Program Companion*.

Training Title: Group Instruction and Inclusion

Purpose

The purpose of this training is to teach trainees to organize activities that teach students to work in small groups and to effectively assist the student in participating in larger groups in included settings.

Target Skills

<u>After completing this training the trainee will be able to:</u>

- Name two general objectives for students participating in group instruction.

- Observe a group activity in a regular preschool or kindergarten and list specific skills required to participate.

- List the *five aspects of the teaching setting* discussed in the chapter and describe how they are manipulated to help a student move from an individualized, discrete trial setting to group instruction.

- Design and conduct an activity similar to the type described in the chapter as a *demonstration/exploration*. Include a list of prerequisite and target skills for the activity.

- Design and conduct an activity similar to the type described in the chapter as a *presentation*. Include a list of basic skills required for participation in the activity.

- State a convenient way to collect data on the target skills listed in the two questions above.

- Name several key factors mentioned that contribute to a successful inclusion experience.

- Name several skills that are important in an inclusion experience.

Reference

Chapter 7: Group Instruction and Inclusion, *The ABA Program Companion.*

Training Title: Creating and Maintaining a Student Schedule

Purpose

The purpose of this training is to teach trainees to create and maintain a student schedule according to established guidelines.

Target Skills

After completing this training the trainee will be able to:

+ Given a blank *Student Schedule Form*, locate the following parts: student name, approximate time of components, component name, boxes that are checked when schedule item is complete, space for date.

+ Given a sample *Student Schedule Form*, fill out a new form for the following week.

+ Given a sample *Student Schedule Form,* mark the form correctly for a given day's activities completed.

Answer the following questions:

+ "Who makes the schedule?" [the consultant, teacher, IA, and other service providers make an initial version of the schedule that is modified and approved by the whole team]

+ "Who reviews the schedule?" [generally, the teacher and the consultant]

+ "True or False – Scheduled component times may *never* be changed." [false]

+ "Name two acceptable reasons why schedule components may be changed, omitted, or added." [e.g., starting new drills and needed to add some repetitions, student is having a difficult day, another drill took longer than expected]

+ "What should you write when you make a change to the schedule?" [describe the change in the check box and on the back of the sheet]

+ "True or False (and explain your answer) – The schedule just lists the drills that are done for the day" [false, the schedule lists all major components of the students curriculum].

+ "Explain the following statement: In a student's schedule there are NO breaks" [There are no breaks in the sense that learning opportunities exist no matter what the

+ student is doing and the teacher needs to continue to present and reinforce good student behavior in all settings]

+ "True or False – When the student is finished with a drill he or she needs a short time away from activities before beginning again" [false—the student may need time in a *different* activity but there should always be opportunities for learning].

Reference

Chapter 8: Organizing an Individualized Curriculum, *The ABA Program Companion.*

Training Title: Orientation to Individual Student Curriculum

Purpose

The purpose of this training is to teach trainees to locate and understand various program documentation materials in preparation for implementing the individual student curriculum and to assist them in participating more effectively in curriculum development.

Target Skills

<u>After attending this training, trainees will be able to:</u>

- List the domains important in establishing a comprehensive curriculum for a young child with autism or PDD.

- Name three settings that should be addressed by any curriculum.

- Referring to a curriculum, state what *sequence and scope* means.

- Name some sources of information in a comprehensive evaluation of a student.

- Describe how curriculum-based assessments are different from other assessment

- Name in the present system, the two processes that comprise the baseline evaluation.

- State where information for the Curriculum Worksheet comes from.

- Discuss how to decide what items from the Curriculum Worksheet should be included on the Probe Data Sheet.

- Describe how the individualized curriculum is organized in the present system. Name the features and format.

- Name some limitations of strictly following normal development in choosing curriculum for a student.

- Discuss how progress is evaluated in the present system including the content of program review meetings.

- State how the Mastered List is used in the present system.

- State what is meant by "there are no breaks in a student schedule."

- Name the sections of the program book and how the sections on curriculum areas are arranged.

<u>With an actual student program book:</u>

- Locate their student's mastered list and list the programs already mastered

- Locate their student's current curriculum and list the programs currently done in each setting.

◈ Locate their student's current schedule (if available) and explain the sequence and timelines of each scheduled component throughout the day.

◈ List several effective reinforcers for their student.

◈ Locate and describe the major procedures in the student's behavior program (if existent).

◈ Locate the Mand List, Tact List, and other natural environment language lists.

◈ Locate and list current play skills and objectives

◈ List important medical or dietary information relevant to the student

Ongoing Training

◈ Read and discuss the behavior program (if existent) with teacher/consultant
◈ Learn to perform all drills (mastered and present) relevant to the student's present curriculum

Reference

Chapter 8: Organizing an Individualized Curriculum, *The ABA Program Companion.*

Chapter 10

PROGRAM EVALUATION

The ability of a program, center, school, or consultant to consistently develop high quality programs depends on many factors including organizational factors, funding, recruitment and training of qualified personnel, staffing ratios, environment, and even less tangible factors like leadership and vision. The New York State Education Department (2001) has promulgated a set of standards in the form of an evaluation checklist called *The Autism Program Quality Indicators* that survey a number of important areas of program function. Yet, at the present time, there is no recognized certification or licensing procedure for ABA programs in existence. Nevertheless, good organizational practices that are recognized to be effective in other types of quality educational programs may also be applied to ABA programs if combined with additional material that surveys practices unique to ABA.

The following program audit is designed primarily for programs with multiple students but can be adapted for use by individual school-based or even home programs. The audit is written to provide a tool to help ensure quality programming by providing specific objective feedback in a variety of areas. It does not necessarily address legal requirements or broader educational licensure standards (e.g., a requirement for a teacher certified in special education or early childhood education). Two general procedures are used to assess compliance with the standards set forth. The *Review of Records and Procedures* is completed by reviewing several individual student records and materials as well as written policies and procedures of the program. Interviews of program personnel may also be used. Indicate the specific method of review and results in the boxes provided. The *Case Review* is completed by directly observing one or more students on several occasions or for a period of time sufficient to obtain stable results from multiple measures. For all parts of the review, the more specific the information and feedback provided, the more helpful.

The audit can be completed by program personnel at various levels within an organization. A program coordinator can complete the audit as a self-initiated review of important program components and as part of a program goal-setting process. However, it is important that periodic impartial review occur by persons not associated with the day-to-day operation of the program in order to objectively identify strong and weak areas.

PROGRAM AUDIT

Part 1: Review of Records and Procedures

Record Keeping and Documentation

Description of Item	Date, Method of Review, and Results
Individual files exist for each student and are immediately accessible to authorized program personnel	
Files contain but are not limited to:	
Contact Information	
Important Medical Information	
Baseline Skills Assessment of appropriate curriculum items that is based on repeated direct measurement	
Copies of all relevant reports from outside consultants and professionals	
Photo and Video Release Permissions if applicable	
Behavior Programs/ authorization for restrictive procedures (if applicable)	
Copies of meeting minutes, letters, and memos concerning student	
Copies of completed (mastered) programs with associated data sheets, stimulus lists, and graphs	
Copies of outdated curriculum with date of revision	

Student Curriculum and Programs

Description of Item	Date, Method of Review, and Results
Individualized student curriculum is comprehensive in scope, appropriate to the age and needs of the student, and reflects continuity with the baseline evaluation.	
The Student's Individualized Curriculum:	
Covers all relevant domains	
Includes behavior program or procedures (if applicable)	
Covers home and community setting support and generalization of skills	
Specifies a variety of teaching settings and includes programs for incidental teaching and inclusion	
Contains comprehensive language program and includes natural environment training as well as work on individual skills in isolation	
The Student's Overall Program:	
Runs for at least 30 hours per week, including summer, without extended periods of vacation or breaks (as required by student need)	
Reviews progress on programs frequently, based on objective measures	
Revises programs in a timely manner if expected progress is not attained	
Is created by an educational team including the parents, teaching personnel, consultant(s), and supporting services such as speech therapy, physical therapy, etc. There is also provision made for participation from the home school district, or parents'	

advisors/representatives as required.	

Program Book

Description of Item	Date, Method of Review, and Results
Separate program book exists for school and home programs (if applicable)	
Sections exist for all curriculum areas	
Program write-ups contain clear descriptions of all procedures, methods, and target behaviors	
Data sheets and stimulus lists exist for all programs and are located with the program write-up	
Mand List, Reinforcer List, and Student Information Sheet exist and are located at the front of the program book	
Student schedule is complete and located in appropriate section of program book	
Student's individualized curriculum exists and is located in a separate section	
Meeting minutes are filed in a separate section of the program book	

Staff and Parent Training

Description of Item	Date, Method of Review, and Results
Training procedures for teaching personnel are described in writing	
Teaching personnel receive training in basic procedures before working with student	
Written training procedures are comprehensive and adequate including trainings in administrative policies, basic methods of applied behavior analysis, basic discrete trial instruction, incidental teaching, language instruction, understanding autism, and the specific program implementation methodologies used by the program.	
Written training procedures exist for training teaching personnel to implement a student's individual curriculum including understanding the program book, student schedule, stimulus lists, data sheets, graphs, mand lists, reinforcer lists, and to understand and participate in the various program review activities (clinics and other meetings).	
Training sessions are documented	
There is written evidence of ongoing professional training for certified teachers in the areas of applied behavior analysis	
There is written evidence of ongoing professional participation and training for consultants	
Written training procedures exist for training parents and other relatives of students in procedures and programs to support the student at home and in the community.	
Procedures exist to orient new parents to the program and program methodology	
There is evidence of regular and effective communication (both formal and informal) between the parents and the program (and school district, if applicable)	
There is evidence that training is offered to relatives on a regular basis according to the needs and schedule of the relatives	
There is evidence of an ongoing outreach to inform and educate	

the neighboring community about effective autism treatment	

Staff Qualifications, Supervision, and Administrative Support

Description of Item	Date, Method of Review, and Results
Instructional Assistants (paraprofessionals) have appropriate experience and training before working with student	
Supervising teacher has experience, education, and professional credentials and certification in areas appropriate to the functioning level, diagnosis, and age of the students	
Supervising teacher has training in all procedures used in the program	
Supervising teacher is familiar with curriculum sequence and scope, as well as mastery criteria for each program	
Supervising teacher is trained in effective supervision techniques and personnel management	
Ratio of students to supervising teacher does not exceed reasonable limits for extended periods of time	
Supervising teacher is scheduled to be on premises for the majority of time	
Consultant(s) and other program supervisors meet the qualifications for Board Certified Behavior Analyst set by the Behavior Analyst Certification Board, Inc.	
Consultant(s) and other program supervisors meet qualifications for ABA consultants in autism set by the Special Interest Group of the Association for Behavior Analysis (1998)	
Formal program review by consultants occurs at least biweekly for each student	
Consultants are easily accessible by phone or other means when they are not present at the program	
Supervising teachers meet individually with paraprofessionals at least biweekly	
Paraprofessionals receive regular objective feedback on their performance, based on direct observation	
All personnel receive written performance reviews at least semi-annually.	
Adequate personnel resources are provided for administrative tasks such as hiring, accounting, and secretarial duties so that programmatic personnel spend time on tasks directly related to accomplishing student goals	
Provision is made for adequately staffing vacancies, illness, vacations, and leaves so that the minimum disruption in programming occurs for the student.	
Input on program goals and services is solicited from community members, parents, and other constituencies	

Environment, Materials, and Equipment

Description of Item	Date, Method of Review, and Results
Environment is large enough to accommodate number of students and adults	
Environment contains sufficient areas for play and other common activities like snack, lunch, and group activities	
Each student has individual space for programs	
Individual student spaces are relatively free from distractions (visual or auditory)	

Individual spaces are not open to view by public	
Environment contains sufficient common space to promote student interaction	
Common areas are readily accessible to student	
Student is regularly allowed access to common space while other students are present	
Environment is free from dirt, unpleasant odors, noise, dangerous equipment, and extremes of temperature	
Electrical outlets are made safe, according to needs of student	
Lighting of area is adequate	
Bathrooms are easily accessible and facilities are easily usable by children (height of sinks, size of toilets, etc.)	
Cleaning supplies are available as needed	
Food storage and preparation is safe.	
Environment contains areas for individual storage of student items	
Students have regular access to outdoors when weather permits	
Outdoor areas are safe and free from dangerous equipment, insects, or animal feces.	
Outdoor areas are well defined and away from vehicles	
Outdoor areas do not permit elopement of students into traffic or other dangerous areas	
Outdoor areas contain sufficient space for all children present to freely engage in gross motor activities	
Outdoor equipment is well maintained and appropriate to the age and developmental level of the children present	
Program possesses equipment and materials to implement all phases of the students' curriculum, including play activities and reinforcement.	
Office and conference areas are separate from programmatic areas	
Area is available for students who are upset to be away from others	
Storage space is sufficient to allow organized access and to keep materials not in use out of the way.	
Materials are clean and disinfected periodically	

Part 2: Case Review

Description of Item	Method of Review
Evaluator completes Teaching Evaluation Checklist on at least two separate occasions for two different students.	Teaching Evaluation Checklist

Student Name: _____ Date and time: _____

Results of Observation 1:

Date and time: _____

Results of Observation 2:

(Attach additional sheets as necessary.)

Part V:
The Consultant's Companion Software for Windows™

Simplify the process of organizing a student's curriculum...

Software that will help your team:

- Print forms for curriculum-based assessment

- Easily choose active goals from hundreds of developmentally sequenced goals organized in major curriculum areas

- Maintain a list of active goals with plenty of space for comments on implementation or progress

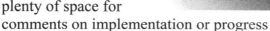
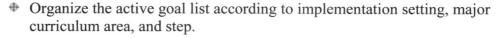

- Organize the active goal list according to implementation setting, major curriculum area, and step.

- Add/modify goals for any area

- Easily print out lists of active and mastered goals

Operation is as simple as:

- Choosing a curriculum area from a drop down menu

- Filling in a setting for each student goal

- Printing out a finished curriculum organized by setting and curriculum area

- **Based on *The Autism Partnership* curriculum in *A Work in Progress* and including over 500 goals in 54 curriculum areas.**

Introduction

Keeping on top of creating and maintaining curriculum goals can be a daunting task for the educational team. A typical curriculum for the ages between birth and three years contains hundreds of goals; the team must choose initial targets in all important domains of functioning, keep track of mastered skills, document discussion and revisions involving individual goals, and make sure that copies of these lists are up to date and available in the master program book. *The Consultant's Companion* software assists teams in getting a handle on the complicated task of curriculum goal control. The software makes it simple to

* Print forms for curriculum-based assessment
* Choose active goals from hundreds of developmentally sequenced goals organized into major curriculum areas
* Maintain a list of currently active goals with space for comments on implementation or progress
* Organize the active goal list according to implementation setting, major curriculum area, and step.
* Add/modify goals for any area
* Print out professionally formatted lists of active and mastered goals

(Please note that a more comprehensive discussion of the process of creating an individualized student curriculum may be found in the preceding chapters.)

Getting Started - Installation

Legal Notice

THE CONSULTANT'S COMPANION
SOFTWARE LICENSE AGREEMENT AND WARRANTY STATEMENT

J. TYLER FOVEL IS WILLING TO LICENSE THE SOFTWARE ONLY UPON THE CONDITION THAT YOU ACCEPT ALL OF THE TERMS CONTAINED IN THIS LICENSE AGREEMENT. PLEASE READ THE TERMS CAREFULLY SINCE STARTING OR CONTINUING TO USE THE SOFTWARE WILL INDICATE YOUR AGREEMENT WITH THE TERMS. IF YOU DO NOT AGREE WITH THESE TERMS, THEN J. TYLER FOVEL IS UNWILLING TO LICENSE THE SOFTWARE TO YOU, IN WHICH EVENT YOU SHOULD DESTROY THE SOFTWARE.

THE SOFTWARE ENTITLED "THE CONSULTANT'S COMPANION, VERSION 1.0 IS A BETA-VERSION OF THE SOFTWARE. THE SOFTWARE IS OFFERED FREE OF CHARGE WITH THE REQUEST THAT USERS PROVIDE THE AUTHOR WITH INFORMATION ON ANY PROBLEMS ENCOUNTERED IN INSTALLATION OR USE. THE AUTHOR WILL USE REASONABLE EFFORTS TO ATTEMPT TO RESOLVE SUCH ISSUES THROUGH EMAIL COMMUNICATIONS BUT NO GUARANTEE IS OFFERED OR IMPLIED THAT ALL PROBLEMS WILL BE RESOLVED. THE AUTHOR PROVIDES THE SOFTWARE "AS-IS." NEITHER J. TYLER FOVEL NOR ANY OF HIS SUPPLIERS MAKES ANY WARRANTY OF ANY KIND, EXPRESS OR IMPLIED. J. TYLER FOVEL AND HIS SUPPLIERS SPECIFICALLY DISCLAIM THE IMPLIED WARRANTEIS OF TITLE, NON-INFRINGEMENT, MERCHANTABILITY, AND FITNESS FOR A PARTICULAR PURPOSE. THERE IS NO WARRANTY OR GUARANTEE THAT THE OPERATION OF THE SOFTWARE WILL BE UNINTERRUPTED, ERROR-FREE, OR VIRUS-FREE, OR THAT THE SOFTWARE WILL MEET ANY PARTICULAR CRITERIA OF PERFORMANCE OR QUALITY. YOU ASSUME THE ENTIRE RISK OF SELECTION, INSTALLATION, AND USE OF THE SOFTWARE. Under local law, certain limitations may not apply, and you may have additional rights which vary from state to state. INDEPENDENT OF THE FOREGOING PROVISIONS, IN NO EVENT AND UNDER NO LEGAL THEORY, INCLUDING WITHOUT LIMITATION, TORT, CONTRACT, OR STRICT PRODUCT LIABILITY, SHALL J. TYLER FOVEL OR ANY OF HIS SUPPLIERS BE LIABLE TO YOU OR ANY OTHER PERSON FOR ANY INDIRECT, SPECIAL, INCIDENTAL, OR CONSEQUENTIAL DAMAGES OF ANY KIND, INCLUDING WITHOUT LIMITATIONS, DAMAGES FOR LOSS OF GOODWILL, WORK STOPPAGE, COMPUTER MALFUNCTION, OR ANY OTHER KIND OF COMMERCIAL DAMAGE, EVEN IF J. TYLER FOVEL HAS BEEN ADVISED OF THE POSSIBILITY OF

Installation Steps

The software will run on Windows 98SE, 2000, ME, and XP. Macintosh versions are not available at this time. System requirements: In addition to the system requirements for the operating systems above, a CD-ROM drive is required for installation, and at least, 20 MB of free hard disk space. An 800x600 display or better is necessary for optimum viewing of screens.

Step 1. Place the accompanying CD in the CD drive and wait a few moments for it to be recognized by the system. Double click on My Computer in the upper left corner of the desktop and then double click on the icon for the CD-ROM drive. Next, double click on the folder marked CCSoftware.

Step 2	
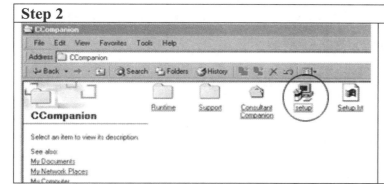	Look for a blue icon of a computer marked SETUP and Double-Click. This will start the installation wizard. The installation process usually takes from 5 – 15 minutes while the files are copied and set up.

Step 3	
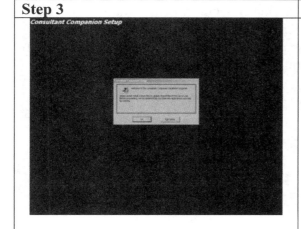	Follow the instructions presented to install the program. The computer may be automatically rebooted several times. The installation wizard will install the program by default at **c:/program files/consultant companion/.** If you decide to change the installation location, **remember this location in order to access the backup function of the program.**

Problems Encountered during Installation

If the computer freezes and there is no hard disk activity for an extended period of time restart the computer and the installation program. NOTE THAT SOME OLDER COMPUTERS MAY BE SLOW IN COPYING FILES so make sure that there is NO HARD DISK ACTIVITY before restarting. If for any other reason, the installation is interrupted, simply run the installation program again. If you encounter any other problems, make sure that no other programs are running such as virus checkers, etc. Shut all extra programs down (except, of course, Windows itself) and run the installation wizard again.

Remember that the program will not install or operate under Windows 95 or 98. If you have an older machine and cannot upgrade to the latest Windows operating system (XP at the time of this writing) try upgrading to Windows 98SE.

If Consultant Companion is not listed on the Program menu or if you still have problems contact the author by email at the address below. If you would like information about software updates and expanded versions of *The Consultant's Companion* send your name and contact information to: tfovel@strategic-alternatives.com. Comments and suggestions are welcome.

Getting Started

Run the program by clicking on the program shortcut found on the Program Menu under Consultant Companion (Start→Programs→Consultant Companion).

Basically, using the program entails adding a student name and then choosing the curriculum items that will be worked on. Assessment information (previously mastered goals) may be added at any time. Once goals are chosen a current curriculum report can be printed. Once assessment information is entered, a mastered list can be printed. For more detailed information on the process of creating an individualized student curriculum see Part III – Planning the Student's Curriculum.

Adding a student

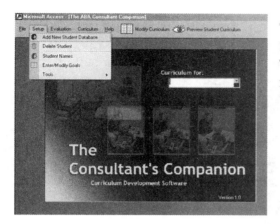

The main screen is pictured at left with the SETUP menu opened to reveal the menu item "Add New Student Database." Click on this item…

…and type in the student's name. Then click the button for Add Name. The dialog box will close. Choose OK when the confirmation box comes up with the student's name.

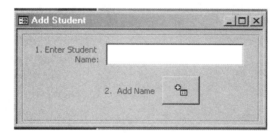

In the main screen locate the pull down menu box under the words "Curriculum for:" Click on the down arrow at the right of the box and choose the new student's name. This is also the way to choose a student curriculum when there is more than one student name entered. (There is no limit on the number of student databases.)

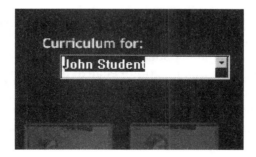

Creating/Modifying an Individualized Student Curriculum

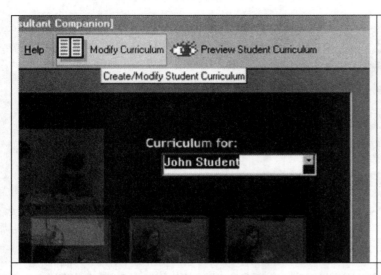

In order to work on the curriculum in any way, you simply click on the button marked "**Modify Curriculum**." You can also click on the menu item listed in the "Curriculum" menu

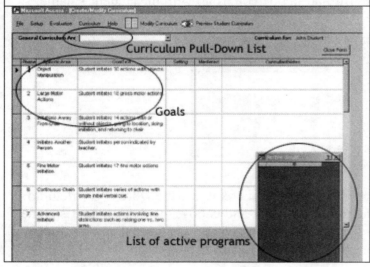

The **Modify Curriculum** form is the main area where you will do your work. Locate the Curriculum Pull-Down List. Clicking on the down arrow will reveal a list of all general curriculum areas. Clicking on an item in the list brings up a list of all program goals under that general area. The goals are listed in general developmental sequence. Each goal is given a title and a description.

Since you have not entered any goals for your new student the **Active Programs** box is blank. Once you choose programs they will be listed in this box according to the general curriculum area. This is a handy snapshot of the student's entire curriculum and is useful when reviewing the items in a meeting because it tells you which curriculum area to go to next without having to refer elsewhere. Note that as you make changes to the curriculum, the active program box does not automatically update itself. If you want to see the changes reflected in the box, close the Modify Curriculum form and reopen it.

Click on the down arrow next to the box marked "General Curriculum Area" and choose an area from the drop-down list. You will see a list of goals corresponding to the area chosen.

Adding Goals to General Curriculum Areas

On the right side of the form a scroll bar is located with up and down arrows click on the down arrow to see additional goals at the bottom of the list. A blank row of boxes is located at the bottom of the goal list for all general curriculum areas. In this row additional goals can be added for a particular student by entering a new phase number, SpecificArea name, and goal text. Any number of new goals can be added. Note that an added goal will apply only to the specific student curriculum that you are working with.

GoalText

Both the title of the skill program (SpecificArea), the text of the goal (GoalText) and the Phase Number are editable. You may change or add text in each of these fields to suit the curriculum needs of the student. For example, you can add a list of specific stimuli on which to work, criteria for advancement, or specific prompts or instructions to use. Note that text for longer goals may be read by clicking in the GoalText field and using the down arrow to scroll down.

Setting

You must enter some sort of text in this area for each item that you want to include in the student's active curriculum. The text can be anything—a word, number, letter—but be aware that it will provide the basis for sorting and printing your active curriculum items. It is recommended that you use descriptors of the setting in which the goal will be implemented. Create a scheme of words that will incorporate all of the settings in which you implement goals, like *drill, home, break, incidental, classroom, gym,* etc. You can use any number of labels but it may be most useful to keep the number down to a few. When printing the active curriculum list, the program will put all of the items with the same descriptor together, starting a new page for each new descriptor. Make sure that you type the descriptors exactly the same, including capitalization.

Mastered

Enter the date of mastery of a goal in this area. You can use any date format that you like. The program will automatically read the format and convert it. If you leave out the year the program will add the current year. Nothing but the date can be entered in this box. The program uses information in this box to keep track of mastered goals according to date and prints the results on the Mastered List. Normally, when starting a new student a complete curriculum evaluation is done for the student and mastery information from this evaluation is entered in this box. The date of the evaluation is usually the date used, indicating that the student had mastered the curriculum goals by this particular date. Entering the evaluation date (baseline date) also can be used to differentiate which goals were mastered before the student started the program vs. which were mastered after starting.

ConsultantNotes

You may enter anything in this box that you wish. It is recommended that you use the area to write short notes about progress or implementation of the goal. Dating each entry will allow you to keep a mini-log of activity on the goal. This area may also be used for listing specific stimuli within programs that are mastered.

Printing Reports

Two reports can be printed based on the information entered in the Modify Curriculum form, the **Mastered List** and the **Curriculum List**.

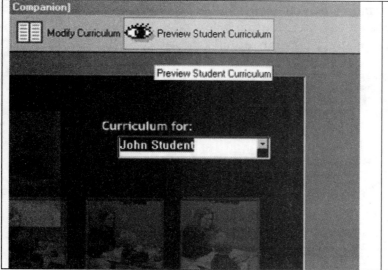

In order to view the Curriculum List onscreen, click on the button marked **"Preview Student Curriculum"** from the main screen.

Sample Curriculum Report

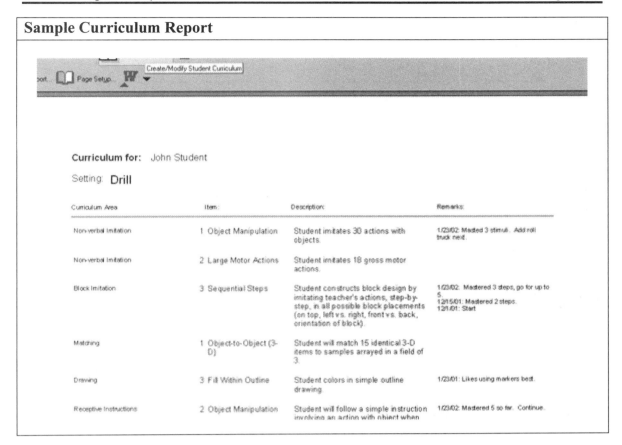

The figure above illustrates part of a Curriculum Report for the setting "Drill." Up-to-date and available curriculum reports are essential for teaching personnel to be able to coordinate their efforts and are an ideal way to provide brief, ongoing guidance on implementation. From the Preview Report screen, you can print any number of copies for distribution and filing. From this screen you can also Export the report as a file, in the word processing format of your choice, Setup the page and printer parameters for printing, or export the report in MS Word format. When you are finished, click the Close button to close the report.

The Mastered List Report

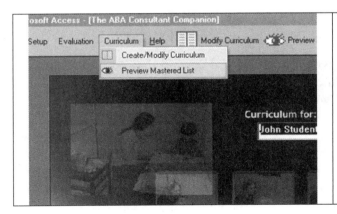

From the main screen menu choose Curriculum and then "Preview Mastered List" to see a formatted list of all items in the curriculum that you have given a date of mastery.

Mastered List: John Student

Goal Number	Curriculum Area	Phase #	Specific Area	Goal	Mastered
24173	Block Imitation	1	Building a Tower	Student builds a tower in response to verbal direction, eight blocks tall.	12/4/2001
24174	Block Imitation	2	Discriminates Colored Shapes	Student matches seven different blocks varying by shape and color to identical sample in a field of three.	12/7/2001
24182	Motor Skills	1	Gross Motor	Student performs 30 gross motor activities	11/4/2001
24204	Drawing	1	Controlling Pen/Scribbling	Student makes mark on paper using pen, crayon, marker in response to Teacher's demonstration and verbal prompt, "Do this."	11/4/2001
24205	Drawing	2	Discriminates Pen Movement	Student marks paper with push/pull strokes and continuous circles when teacher demonstrates and says, "Do this."	12/14/2001
24215	Play	1	Solitary Play	Student will play Pat-a-Cake	10/4/2001

The Mastered List is organized by curriculum area of the program. It displays the name of the curriculum area the phase or step of the program, the name of the program, a description of the program, and the date mastered. As with the Curriculum Report the Preview Screen allows printing and exporting of the report.

Evaluation Forms

Two types of curriculum-based evaluation forms can be printed. The first is called the Curriculum Worksheet. It is a list of all goals in the current curriculum master database arranged according to general curriculum area. This list can be filled out by those who know the student well as an initial report of a student's skills with respect to the curriculum. Access this form from the Evaluation menu (Preview Curriculum Worksheet).

The second form available is called the Probe Data Sheet. This form is created by typing the word "Probe" in the Setting field of the Create/Modify Curriculum form for a number of goals. The goals chosen form the initial data-based *baseline evaluation* and the form includes boxes for the notation of data collected. A more complete discussion of the use of this form is included in the discussion following these instructions.

Additional Features

Deleting a Student Database

CAUTION: This operation is irreversible and will delete all data for a student form the database. From the Setup menu choose Delete Student. Choose the name of the student to be deleted from the pull-down menu and click Delete Student Data.

Editing Student Names

If you inadvertently misspell the name of a student or want to change a name choose Student Names from the Setup menu. Choose the name that you would like to change from the pull down menu on the left and enter the new name in the text box on the right. Complete the change by clicking on the button Make Name Change. If you change your mind you can dismiss the box without making any changes by clicking on the X (close) box in the top right corner.

Backing up Student Data

It is important to regularly back up your data. Computer files can become damaged or hard drives can crash. If you accepted the defaults during installation, a file called **backup.mdb** was created at location **c:/program files/ccompanion/**. If you installed the program in another location you will need to remember that location. From the Setup menu of the program choose Tools and then Backup Student Data. Use the dialogue box to navigate to the backup location. Highlight the file **backup.mdb** and click on Export All to save the first table (Student Data). A dialogue box will appear that says, "Export Student IEP Goals to Student IEP Goals…" Click OK. A new dialogue box will appear that says, "The database object 'Student IEP Goals' already exists. Do you want to replace…" Click on YES. Next a dialogue box will come up to save the second table (Student Names). Again find the backup.mdb file and highlight it. Then click Export All and OK to the next dialogue box that says "Export Student Info…" Finally, answer YES to the next box which says "The database object 'Student Info' already exists…" to complete the process of backup.

Restoring Files

From the Setup menu choose Tools and then Restore Student Data. Follow instructions given in the dialogue box to complete the restore process.

Adding and Deleting Goals in a Curriculum

Goals may be added or deleted from the curriculum of an individual student or to the master goal list. Note that if you add or delete goals from the master goal list this will only be effective for *future* added students, *not* students already added.

You **add** goals to individual student curriculums in the Create/Modify Curriculum form. Simply go to the general curriculum area where you will put the new goal. Scroll to the bottom of the list of goals to find a blank row and enter the information for the new goal: phase number, specific area, and goal text.

Goals may be easily **deleted** from the same Create/Modify Curriculum form by placing the cursor in the area of the screen to the left of the phase number in the row of the goal to be deleted. The cursor will change to a right arrow. Click in the space to highlight the row and press the Delete key. Confirm the deletion by choosing OK.

If you would like to add goals to the master goal list you can also create new general curriculum areas. From the Setup menu choose Enter/Modify Goals and complete the fields for each goal.

Compacting and Repairing Database

Use this utility occasionally to keep the file size of your student database as small as possible. From the Setup menu choose Tools and then Compacting and Repairing Database.

Registering the Software

If you would like to be informed of future software updates and improvements or other training materials that may become available send your contact information to the author at:

Strategic Alternatives
Tyler Fovel
15 Deerfield Road
Medway, MA 02053

Or via email to:
tfovel@strategic-alternatives.com

Please print legibly:

Name: _____

Address: Street: _____

                Town: _____ State: _____ Zip: _____

Email: _____

Date Purchased: _____

Place Purchased: _____   Version: Beta

Thank you for using The Consultant's Companion software.

Appendix

The following forms may be copied for clinical purposes as long as the copyright notice is not removed.

Contents:

Teaching Evaluation Checklist
Typical Instructions for Preschoolers and Kindergarteners
Discrete trials data sheet
Stimulus list
Mand list
Potential reinforcer list
Student schedule form
Incidental language data sheet
Incidental teaching form
Probe Data Sheet
Curriculum Form
Mastered List Form

Teaching Evaluation Checklist

Therapist: _____   Evaluator: _____

Date _____   Setting: _____

Structure /Setup/Environmental	Occurred	Did Not Occur	N/A
Materials ready / organized before session			
Unnecessary distracters removed			
Reinforcers and materials kept accessible			
Therapist follows schedule			
Therapist sits at optimal distance / position			

Comments (continued on back):

Discrete Trial Programs	Occurred	Did Not Occur	N/A
Therapist established attention before giving instruction			
Instructions clear and discriminable			
Instructions given without interruption			
Instructions/materials presented in a fluid manner			
Instruction is brief, specific and as prescribed			
Stimuli presented from stimulus list			
Inter-trial intervals were appropriate length. Pacing was appropriate to maximize motivation and interest.			
Data recorded during inter-trial interval			
Prompts used only as needed			
Prompts were used effectively			
Prompts delivered in appropriate amount of time			
Therapist used all opportunities for incidental teaching (e.g., language)			
Error correction procedure followed when necessary			

Comments (continued on back):

Teaching Evaluation Checklist

Therapist:_____

Reinforcement / Motivation system	Occurred	Did Not Occur	N/A
Reinforcements were effective/appropriate for student			
Edibles were appropriately prepared/delivered			
Reinforcers were delivered contingent upon correct responses, attending, and lack of inappropriate behavior			
Therapist reinforced responses that were closest to the desired response			
Therapist voice and demeanor was clearly reinforcing			
Reinforcers were paired with behavior-specific praise			
Therapist varied reinforcers			
Comments (continued on back):			

Behavior Reduction Programs	Occurred	Did Not Occur	N/A
1. Treatment of behavior (s) as specified in treatment programs			
2. Therapist took appropriate data			
3. Therapist used appropriate differential reinforcement			
4. Therapist interrupted activities to gain instructional control and re-establish program when child was attending			
5. Therapist redirected and/or ignored behaviors that have no specific intervention(s).			
Comments (continued on back):			

Teaching Evaluation Checklist

Page 3   **Therapist:**_____

Incidental Teaching	Occurred	Did Not Occur	N/A
Therapist prompted / provided opportunities for appropriate play / "free time" activities			
Therapist prompted activities from curriculum			
Activities were appropriate to the skill level of child			
Therapist utilized opportunities to facilitate language			
Therapist facilitated independence with activities			
Therapist gave student appropriate amount of "free play"			
Comments			

Adapted from a checklist by Jill McGrale, used with permission

Summary Comments

Typical Worksheet Instructions for Preschool and Kindergarten

- Color each picture red
- Color the _____ red
- Color the one that is different red
- Color the one that is the same red
- Circle the blue picture in each row
- Draw a picture of something else green
- Color the picture
- Color each picture the same color as the crayon above it
- Color the fruits and vegetables
- Cut out the shapes and glue them in the correct color box
- Trace the circle below. Then draw a line under the circle in each row.
- Circles can be different sizes. Trace the circles below. Then color the pictures.
- Draw an X on the pictures that have the shape of a circle.
- Squares have four sides of the same length. Help Sue get home. Color the path that has only squares.
- Trace and color each shape. Draw and color two more of each shape.
- Look at the shapes in the picture. Color the circles blue. Color the squares red. Color the triangles green.
- Cut out the shapes and glue them on paper to make a picture
- Help Jim get to the kite shop. Color the path that has only diamonds.
- Draw a line to the matching pictures
- Trace the star below. Then draw a line under the star in each row.
- Connect the dots in order to make your own stars.
- Color the stars. How many stars?
- Look at the shapes. How many white shapes? How many blue stars?
- Draw a line from each shape to the basket it belongs in.
- Bob is looking for stars. Help him find them. Color all the stars blue.
- Listen to the riddle and tell me the answer:
    - I can move
    - You can ride in me
    - I have four circles
    - My seat belts keep you safe
    - What am I?
- Draw an X on the shapes in each row that are different from the first shape
- Color the shape in each row that looks the same as the first shape
- Draw an X on the picture in each box that is different
- Color the pictures in each row that go together. Draw an X on the one that does not belong.
- Cut out the boxes below. Match the pictures that go together.
- Opposites are things that are different in every way. Draw a line to match the opposites
- Draw a picture of the opposite
- Look at the pictures in each box. Circle the pictures that are big.
- Look at the pictures in each box. Circle the pictures that are small.
- Color the small pictures in each box orange. Color the big pictures purple
- Cut out the boxes below. Put the animals in order from smallest to biggest
- Circle the thing in each box that is long.
- Circle the thing in each box that is short
- Circle the picture in each box that has something short
- Cut out the measuring stick at the bottom of the page. Measure each pencil below. How many boxes long is this pencil?
- Draw an X on the shorter pencil. Circle the longer pencil
- Use the measuring stick from page 90 to measure these pencils
- Circle the picture that is taller. Draw an X on the picture that is shorter.
- Circle the full container. Draw an X on the empty container
- Look at the picture. The sun is above the bird. Circle the pictures above the bird.

Typical Worksheet Instructions for Preschool and Kindergarten

P. 2

o   Look at the picture. The car is below the bird. Draw an X on the pictures below the bird.
o   Circle the picture that is above the others. Draw an X on the picture that is below the others.
o   Color the pictures above the clouds first. Then color the pictures below the clouds
o   Trace and color the cat that is between the other cats. Color the mouse that is between the other mice.
o   Color the shape that is between the other shapes
o   Draw a line from the top picture to the bottom picture
o   Color the pictures on the left blue. Color the pictures on the right red.
o   Draw a line from the picture on the left to the picture on the right
o   Names are special. We use capital letters to set them apart from other words. Circle the capital letters in the names below.
o   Write your name. Circle the capital letter.
o   Write your name. Draw a picture of yourself doing something you like.
o   Write your house number on the house.
o   Write your address. Draw a picture to show where you live.
o   Write your phone number. Practice dialing it using the phone below.
o   Trace and write the letter A. Start at the dot. Say the sound the letter makes as you write it.
o   Circle the letters in each row that match the first letter.
o   Look at the letter each insect is holding. Circle the same letter below.
o   Trace and write the letter D. Start at the dot. Say the sound the letter makes as you write it.
o   Look at the uppercase letter in each row. Color each picture with a matching lowercase letter.
o   Draw a line from each uppercase letter to its matching lowercase letter
o   Help the walrus get back to the sea by following the letters in ABC order
o   Find out what the elves are making. Draw a line to connect the dots in ABC order
o   Draw a line from each uppercase letter to its matching lowercase letter. Then color the pictures.
o   Help Adam get to the playground. Follow the letters in ABC order.
o   Color each fish that has an uppercase and lowercase letter that match
o   Color all the letters red. Color all the numbers blue. Write the letter message below.
o   Color the spaces with the J sound blue. Color the other spaces yellow.
o   Help the birds find their nest. Follow the path with the pictures whose names begin with the same sound as nest.
o   Short Oo is the sound at the beginning of the word octopus. Say each picture name. Color the socks that have the short Oo sound. Does this octopus have enough colored socks?
o   Say each picture name. Say each word. Draw a line from each picture to the word that names the picture.
o   Say each picture name. Cut out the words. Glue each word where it belongs.
o   Say the sound the letters make. Circle the pictures in each row that begin with the letter shown.
o   Pam only picks things whose names begin with the same sound as panda. Say the picture names. Circle each picture whose name begins with the same sound as Pam and Panda.
o   Look at the pictures on the quilt below. Say each picture name. If the picture begins with the same sound as quilt, color the square yellow. Color the other squares purple.
o   Look at the letter in each column. Cut out each picture and glue it under the correct beginning sound

DATA COLLECTION

Curriculum Area:

Step Name:

STUDENT:

| + | = CORRECT | — | = INCORRECT | P | = PROMPTED | I | = INDEPENDENT |

Instruction:

Date/Initials	1	2	3	4	5	6	7	8	9	10	11	12	13	14	15	SCORE (%)

STIMULUS LIST

General Area: _____   **Program Name:** _____

Instruction: _____

Stimulus Or Step	Added as new performance (practiced with prompts)	In Random Rotation	Date Mastered in Random Rotation	Generalization – Locations		Generalization – People		Generalization – Instructions	
				✓	M	✓	M	✓	M

MAND LIST

Student: _____   Date Started: _____

Date Added	Stimulus Conditions	Mand
	In these circumstances: (example: when student approaches or touches TV.)	**Indicate word(s) or describe actions** (example: "T.V." or Signs TV or Points to picture of TV)

Use additional pages as necessary

POTENTIAL REINFORCER LIST

Student: _____   **Date Started:**_____

EDIBLES	SOCIAL	TOYS	ACTIVITES	GAMES	OTHER

STUDENT SCHEDULE

Student: _____   Date:_____

APPROX. TIME:	SCHEDULE COMPONENT/DRILL	DAY (✔ if completed)				
		MON	TUES	WED	THU	FRI

(COMMENTS ON BACK)

Incidental Language Data Sheet

Student Behavior
M = Mands
T = Tacts
VI = Verbal Imitation
I = Intraverbal
VOC = Vocalization (not word)
J = Jargon/Echolalia

Antecedents (choose one)
S = Spontaneous
VP = Verbally Prompted
CT = Communication Temptation Created by Teacher

Consequences: (note all that are delivered)
IG = Purposely Ignored to Encourage Closer Approximation
R = Model Prompt Given to Refine Pronunciation
L = Longer Utterance Required
R+ = Reinforced by teacher

Instructions: categorize each utterance of the student using the labels above and write the code in the first blank box below marked "student" (working downwards). For each student utterance choose the antecedent and consequences observed from the list above and write the code in the corresponding boxes

Date: _____ Instructor: _____

Location/Activity: _____

Start Time: _____ End Time: _____ Observer: _____

Antecedent	Student Behavior	Consequences	Antecedent	Student Behavior	Consequences

Incidental Teaching Curriculum List

Student: _____ **Date:** _____ **Page:** _____

Setting/Activity	Category	Current Target Behaviors:
	Primary Skills	
	Incidental Skills	
	Primary Skills	
	Incidental Skills	
	Primary Skills	
	Incidental Skills	
	Primary Skills	
	Incidental Skills	

Data Sheet

Probe Programs for: _____

Setting: _____

Curriculum Area	Program Name	Description of Goal	Data & Date							

Use back of form for additional space

Curriculum for: _____

Date: _____

Setting: _____

Page _____ **of** _____

Curriculum Area	Program Name	Description of Goal	Consultant Notes

Mastered List for: _____

Date: _____

Page _____ of _____

Curriculum Area	Step/ Phase #	Specific Program Name	Description of Goal	Mastery Date